Quality of Life in Asia

Volume 11

This series, the first of its kind, examine both the objective and subjective dimensions of life quality in Asia, especially East Asia. It unravels and compares the contours, dynamics and patterns of building nations, offering innovative works that discuss basic and applied research, emphasizing inter- and multi-disciplinary approaches to the various domains of life quality. Thus, the series appeals to a variety of fields in humanities, social sciences and other professional disciplines. Asia is the largest, most populous continent on Earth, and it is home to the world's most dynamic region, East Asia. In the past three decades, East Asia has been the most successful region in the world in expanding its economies and integrating them into the global economy, offering lessons on how poor countries, even with limited natural resources, can achieve rapid economic development. Yet while scholars and policymakers have focused on why East Asia has prospered, little has been written on how its economic expansion has affected the quality of life of its citizens. The series publish several volumes a year, either single or multipleauthored monographs or collections of essays.

More information about this series at http://www.springer.com/series/8416

Yuet Wah Cheung • Nicole Wai-ting Cheung

Psychoactive Drug Abuse in Hong Kong

Life Satisfaction and Drug Use

Springer

Yuet Wah Cheung
Department of Sociology
Hong Kong Shue Yan University
Hong Kong, China

Nicole Wai-ting Cheung
Department of Sociology
The Chinese University of Hong Kong
Hong Kong, China

ISSN 2211-0550 ISSN 2211-0569 (electronic)
Quality of Life in Asia
ISBN 978-981-13-5583-7 ISBN 978-981-10-6154-7 (eBook)
DOI 10.1007/978-981-10-6154-7

Printed on acid-free paper

This Springer imprint is published by Springer Nature
The registered company is Springer Nature Singapore Pte Ltd.
The registered company address is: 152 Beach Road, #21-01/04 Gateway East, Singapore 189721, Singapore

Preface

This book is an in-depth analysis of the data of the "Longitudinal Survey of Psychoactive Drug Abusers in Hong Kong" (LSPDA). Conducted during 2009–2012 and funded by the Beat Drugs Fund established by the government, the 3-year longitudinal study was the first of its kind in Hong Kong, tackling the alleged social problem of soaring prevalence of psychoactive drug use in young people since the mid-1990s (for the report of the study, see Cheung Y.W. (2012). *A longitudinal survey of psychoactive drug abusers in Hong Kong*. Report submitted to Narcotics Division, Government of the Hong Kong SAR.). Ketamine stood out as the most popular psychoactive drug since 2000. This had caught youth drug workers, medical and legal professionals, teachers, parents, community leaders, and government officials by surprise, as ketamine was not a widely used drug worldwide and at that time little was known about the drug's pharmacological properties other than its use as an anaesthesia in animal surgical operations.

Medical research on the physical and mental harm of ketamine abuse had to quickly begin in the early 2000s in order to acquire more knowledge of the properties of ketamine, badly needed for the design of appropriate treatment and prevention strategies. However, large-scale social scientific studies of the characteristics of ketamine users and factors influencing their ketamine use were seriously lacking. LSPDA filled this research gap by studying a sample of ketamine users recruited from youth outreach agencies and treatment programmes. This book offers a comprehensive analysis of the data of LSPDA, focusing on the socio-demographic and psychosocial correlates of ketamine use in young psychoactive drug users. Practical implications for treatment and prevention efforts are also discussed.

Incidentally, the senior author had conducted a longitudinal study of drug abusers in Hong Kong some 10 years before LSPDA. That study was entitled "Longitudinal Study of Chronic Drug Abusers in Hong Kong" (LSCDA), conducted from 2000 to 2003 and also funded by the Beat Drugs Fund (for the report, see Cheung Y.W. (2003). *A longitudinal study of chronic drug abusers in Hong Kong*. Report submitted to Narcotics Division, Government of the Hong Kong SAR; for the subsequent book, see Cheung Y.W. (2009). *A brighter side: Protective and risk factors in the rehabilitation of chronic drug abusers in Hong Kong*. Hong Kong:

Chinese University Press.). At that time, although young people's psychoactive drug use had begun to pop up, the majority of drug abusers were still adults addicted to heroin, the conventional drug of choice in Hong Kong for many decades. A large number of socio-demographic and psychosocial variables were introduced in the study to gauge the protective and risk factors of post-treatment drug use among chronic heroin abusers. This earlier longitudinal study (LSCDA) addressed an older generation of users of heroin; 10 years later, LSPDA examined the younger generation of users of ketamine and other psychoactive drugs. These two landmark studies echoed each other, and together they captured the major changes in drug abuse patterns and their psychosocial correlates across the two generations.

Among the psychosocial variables used in the two longitudinal studies to explain continuation/discontinuation of drug use, one of them—life satisfaction—was included in both studies. Life satisfaction was found to be significantly related to drug use in both studies, after controlling for other psychosocial variables. This is perhaps the first evidence showing the importance of life satisfaction in affecting drug use among drug abusers of both generations in Hong Kong. It is a tempting invitation to a more elaborate exploration of the role of quality of life in the prevalence of young people's psychoactive drug use, as well as the design of relevant treatment strategies. This has become the major objective of this book, which is based on LSPDA. In the multivariate analysis, the effect of life satisfaction on the continuation/discontinuation of drug use of psychoactive drug users is compared with those of other important psychosocial variables, such as permissiveness to drug use (derived from the normalization of recreational drug use perspective), self-esteem, depression, stressful life events, experience of discrimination, and sense of uncertainty about the future. Gender differences in how life satisfaction and other psychosocial variables had influenced drug use are also examined. In addition, a chapter is devoted to the discussion of the role of subjective well-being in the treatment and rehabilitation of psychoactive drug addiction. It is hoped that this unique analysis will serve as a springboard for more fruitful research on this topic in the future.

We owe the idea of publishing this book to Professor Daniel T.L. Shek of Hong Kong Polytechnic University, who saw the potential of an in-depth analysis of the data of LSPDA in contributing to the scanty literature of life satisfaction and drug use/drug treatment in Hong Kong. Without his encouragement and patience, we would not have finished the manuscript. Dr. Celia X. Chen and Ms. Cherry Y.T. Choi had provided us with valuable assistance in data analysis. The Narcotics Division kindly gave us the permission to use the data of LSPDA. We would also like to express our great appreciation to those treatment and rehabilitation agencies that had actively participated in the survey for 3 years, without which this study would not have been successfully conducted.

Hong Kong, China

Yuet Wah Cheung
Nicole Wai-ting Cheung

The original version of the Index was revised. The version supplied here includes final author corrections.

Chapter 1
Changes of the Drug Scene in Hong Kong

From Heroin to Psychoactive Drugs

Heroin has been on the centre stage of the drug scene in Hong Kong for many decades, due mainly to the legacy of opium in Hong Kong. Opium was used by Britain as its major item of trade with China during the Qing Dynasty in the nineteenth century. Confronted with Western gunboats, the feeble China suffered numerous losses and setbacks in its conflicts with Western powers forcing trade to this "Middle Kingdom". After losing two Opium Wars to the British (1839–1842, 1856–1860), and in another Sino-British conflict in 1898, parts of Hong Kong were either ceded or leased for 99 years to the British (Hsü 1995). The sovereignty of the whole of Hong Kong was reverted to the present Chinese regime in 1997.

After Hong Kong became a British colony in the mid-nineteenth century, the British Hong Kong government maintained a monopoly in the sale and distribution of opium, thereby generating large tax revenues (Traver 1992). Since the early twentieth century, there had been escalating international pressures on Britain to stop the sale of opium in its colonies. In 1945, opium was finally listed in the Dangerous Drugs Ordinance and became an illicit drug in Hong Kong. The drug policy of Hong Kong then changed from "monopoly" to "prohibition" (Cheung and Ch'ien 1996). Heroin, a derivative of opium, had then become increasingly popular since the early twentieth century. Compared with opium, heroin had a relative advantage because it was in powder form and was more convenient to carry, more profitable, and easier to administer use. Since the 1950s, heroin had dominated the illicit drug scene in Hong Kong for decades.

The dominance of heroin in Hong Kong's drug scene can be reflected by the data of Central Registry of Drug Abuse (CRDA[1]), a database maintained by the Narcotics

[1] The Central Registry of Drug Abuse (CRDA) is a database established in 1972 by the Narcotics Division for the collection of drug abuse statistics that are useful for monitoring drug abuse trends and understanding the characteristics of drug abusers. Through a voluntary reporting system, CRDA collates information of drug abusers submitted by reporting organizations in drug treat-

Y.W. Cheung, N.W.-t. Cheung, *Psychoactive Drug Abuse in Hong Kong*,
Quality of Life in Asia 11, DOI 10.1007/978-981-10-6154-7_1

Table 1.1 All reported individuals reported to CRDA by primary drug of abuse

September 1976 – December 1981						
Selected type of drugs (%)	1976	1977	1978	1979	1980	1981
Heroin	82.4	85.7	89.5	93.9	93.8	95.3
Opium	11.1	11.5	5.9	4.0	3.2	2.5
Other narcotics	5.9	2.6	4.4	1.9	2.7	1.7
Non-narcotics	0.6	0.2	0.2	0.2	0.3	0.5
No. of individuals	6755	10154	6280	3862	2507	1650

Source: *CRDA Ninth Report* (Narcotics Division 1982)

Division of the government, to which drug treatment, health care, law enforcement, and social service organizations voluntarily submit information of their clients found to be drug users. An example is found in the ninth report of CRDA (Narcotics Division 1982), which shows the percentages of reported individuals whose primary drugs of abuse were heroin, opium, other narcotics, or non-narcotics for the period from September 1976 to December 1981 (Table 1.1).

In Table 1.1, it can be seen that over 99% of reported individuals for the years concerned were narcotics users. The percentages of non-narcotics users ranged from 0.2 to 1.6% only. Among narcotics users, heroin was their primary drug of abuse. As CRDA only contains data pertaining to users reported to drug, health, law enforcement, and social service agencies, it does not include users who do not fall into the locus of these agencies. Despite this limitation, the overwhelming choice of heroin before the 1980s was obvious.

While heroin has been the most dominant drug, psychoactive drugs have never been absent from the drug scene of Hong Kong. Psychoactive drugs often refer to mood-altering drugs (Cheung 2000:1697). In Hong Kong, a similar term – "psychotropic substances" – is traditionally used by the government to describe drugs that affect a person's mental activity and perception. In the classification of illicit drugs by the Narcotics Division, substances of abuse are broadly divided into two categories (Narcotics Division 2014). The first category is "narcotics analgesics", including heroin, opium, morphine, and physeptone/methadone. The second category is "psychotropic substances", which include hallucinogens (e.g. cannabis, LSD), depressants (barbiturates, methaqualone, GSB), stimulants (e.g. amphetamines, cocaine, MDMA), tranquillizers (e.g. benzodiazepines), and other substances (e.g. ketamine, mephedrone, cough medicine, alcohol, tobacco, organic solvents). Such

ment, medical and health service, law enforcement, and social welfare services (Narcotics Division 2014). The confidentiality of information of CRDA is legally protected and is not accessible without a court order. There are two major weaknesses of this database. First, the information obtained cannot include drug users who are not in contact with reporting organizations and thus not reported. Second, there is a tendency for some organizations to be more willing than others to report cases. For example, law enforcement agencies would be more willing to report cases than social service organizations whose social workers would have the concern that if their drug-using clients know that they are reported, then the rapport with their clients might be undermined (Cheung and Ch'ien 1996).

a classification scheme is so broad that it practically includes all those drugs that do not belong to the narcotics category.

Multiple drug use is a very common practice among drug users worldwide, and so even though heroin was the most popular drug in Hong Kong, non-narcotic drugs such as cannabis, amphetamine, and cocaine, currently placed under the category of psychotropic drugs in Narcotics Division's classification scheme, must have also been simultaneously used. However, there had not been any particular psychotropic drug that could challenge the dominance of heroin, until the late 1990s, when young drug users started to break away from heroin and turn to psychoactive drugs, especially new ones. Table 1.2 captures this new phenomenon.

Table 1.2 gives information on the use of heroin and selected psychoactive drugs by CRDA reported individuals who were under the age of 21, as well as the use of heroin and ketamine, one of the most recent psychoactive drugs, among individuals aged 21 or over, during the period from 1980 to 2013. The first thing to note is the percentage of reported individuals aged under 21 who had used heroin (first row of Table 1.2). In the early 1980s, this group of users was still overwhelmingly using heroin. Their percentage of having used heroin was 97.7% in 1980, 94.4% in 1982, 94.3% in 1984, and 80.9% in 1986. This percentage began to drop since the late 1980s, as only 59.1% of this group of reported individuals had used heroin in 1988. In the following decade, the percentage of heroin users fluctuated but did not rebound to over 80%. An even sharper decline occurred in 2000, when the percentage dropped to only 21.6%, followed by continuous decrease to less than 6% from 2006 onwards.

At the same time, the rapid rise in psychoactive drug use among reported individuals aged under 21 since the late 1990s has been noteworthy (see Table 1.2). The percentage of reported individuals of this age group having used methamphetamine (ice) rose from 7.6% in 1996 to 41% in 2015. The percentage having used cannabis increased sharply from 4.1% in 1986 to 24.7% in 1988 and remained mostly over 20% from 1990 to 2004, before dropping to around 10% until 2015. Cocaine registered its presence in this age group in 2002 and rose quickly from 0.6% in that year to 9.4% in 2008 and 27.5% in 2015. Abuse of cough medicine also experienced a sharp increase from 2.9% in 1988 to 25.3% in 1992, before dropping to less than 10% in the following years, due to the implementation of the requirement of purchase with a doctor's prescription in mid-1990s. Ecstasy (MDMA), a newly popular drug among young people consumed especially in discos and large-scale rave parties since the late 1990s, had attracted 56.2% of reported individuals under 21 in 2000. As rave parties began to decline since the mid-2000s, the percentage of this age group of users having used ecstasy quickly dropped to 15.6% in 2008 and then to only 1.8% in 2012.

But the most staggering phenomenon is the sharp landing of ketamine on the drug scene in the late 1990s. Primarily used as a horse tranquillizer since decades ago, ketamine use did not appear in CRDA data until 2000, when suddenly more than one-third (36.9%) of reported individuals aged under 21 had used it. This percentage continued to rise very quickly, almost doubling itself in 2002 (70.5%), and

Table 1.2 Reported (newly and previously) individuals aged "under 21" and "21 and over" by selected type of drugs abused

Selected type of drug	1980 (%)	1982 (%)	1984 (%)	1986 (%)	1988 (%)	1990 (%)	1992 (%)	1994 (%)	1996 (%)	1998 (%)	2000 (%)	2002 (%)	2004 (%)	2006 (%)	2008 (%)	2010 (%)	2012 (%)	2014 (%)	2015 (%)
Aged under 21																			
Heroin	97.7	94.4	94.3	80.9	59.1	48.2	58.0	79.5	66.6	58.4	21.6	10.7	5.3	2.0	1.8	2.8	4.8	5.2	5.9
Ketamine	–	–	–	–	–	–	–	–	–	–	36.9	70.5	69.6	73.5	85.5	80.1	61.1	46.6	38.5
Ecstasy	–	–	–	–	–	–	–	–	<.05	2.0	56.2	37.1	38.3	42.6	15.6	5.8	1.8	-	-
Methamphetamine (Ice)	–	–	–	–	–	–	–	–	7.6	17.3	11.0	8.1	6.7	10.3	14.9	21.9	30.1	38.5	41.0
Cannabis	–	0.8	0.7	4.1	24.7	29.5	22.9	17.9	21.0	26.6	21.2	25.8	25.5	18.6	9.0	8.0	8.7	10.6	11.2
Cocaine	—	–	–	–	–	–	–	–	–	–	–	0.6	0.9	6.7	9.4	15.3	23.7	24.6	27.5
Cough medicine	–	–	–	–	2.9	15.7	25.3	11.0	7.8	5.2	2.6	3.0	9.6	6.9	3.1	2.7	4.0	2.9	2.6
No of individuals under 21 with known type of drug reported	516	735	971	787	697	892	1653	3891	3363	2551	3466	2490	2127	2551	3464	2799	1592	805	659
% of individuals aged under 21 among reported individuals of all age groups with known type of drug reported	4.2	6.2	7.9	8.1	6.0	6.6	12.1	20.1	18.1	16.2	21.1	15.6	14.6	19.4	24.4	22.4	14.4	9.0	7.8
Aged 21 and over																			
Heroin	93.9	96.4	98.2	98.0	97.5	95.9	96.5	96.2	90.8	91.7	88.3	86.0	80.9	75.9	66.9	63.2	60.9	56.0	55.4
Ketamine	–	–	–	–	–	–	–	–	–	–	2.5	7.0	8.9	11.3	19.9	23.9	24.6	22.6	21.9

Source: Central Registry of Drug Abuse, 25th, 36th, 56th and 64th Reports (Narcotics Division)
– No reported information

reaching its peak of 85.5% in 2008, before starting to decrease from 2010 onwards (80.1% in 2010, 61.1% in 2012, and 38.5% in 2015).

Throughout the past 15 years, as the age of young ketamine users increased, the percentage of reported individuals aged 21 or over having used ketamine also began to increase since the early 2000s, from 2.5% in 2000 to 21.9% in 2015. Concomitantly, the percentage of these adult users having used heroin started to drop from 88.3% in 2000 to 55.4% in 2015 (see the last two rows in Table 1.2).

The seriousness of the problem of psychoactive drug abuse among young people was reflected not only by the sudden popularity of ketamine, ecstasy, and other psychoactive drugs among young people; the sharp increase in the number of reported individuals under 21 having taken one or more illicit drugs also sent a great alarm to the public and the government. In Table 1.2, this number was only 516 in 1980 but rose to 892 in 1990 and hit 3891 in 1994. The number fluctuated but still stood at 3464 in 2008, before dropping to 659 in 2015.

The percentage of reported individuals aged under 21 among reported individuals of all age groups also tells the same story. Before 1990, only less than 10% of all reported individuals were under the age of 21, but this percentage almost doubled itself from 6.6% in 1990 to 12.1% in 1992 and continued to rise to 24.4% in 2008 before dropping to 7.8% in 2015 (Table 1.2).

When the alarming increase of young people's drug use first appeared in the early 1990s, the then Governor of Hong Kong, Mr. Chris Patten, held two drug summits in 1995 and 1996, respectively, to bring together an array of legal and medical professionals, service providers, academics, and teachers to discuss the best strategy to tackle the problem (Cheung 1998). The summits resulted in the government's stronger commitment of resources and coordinating efforts to various aspects of drug work. The Beat Drugs Fund was established in 1996 with the purpose of providing extra funding to sponsor new and worthwhile projects in treatment and rehabilitation, prevention and education, and research (Narcotics Division 2017a). The new tide of drug use among young people that arrived in the early 2000s once again caught the attention of the public. As the prevalence of use of psychoactive drugs, especially ketamine, by young people continued to rise, the then Chief Executive, Mr. Donald Tsang, established an interdepartmental Task Force on Youth Drug Abuse, led by the Secretary for Justice, in 2007 to tackle the problem of psychoactive drug abuse in young people (Task Force on Youth Drug Abuse 2008). A voluntary Trial Scheme on School Drug Testing was implemented in secondary schools in the Tai Po District from 2009 to 2010 and then extended to 2010–2011 (Narcotics Division 2011). The preventive and deterrence functions of the scheme were positively evaluated, leading to the implementation of the Healthy School Programme, which incorporated voluntary drug test and anti-drug preventive education activities in secondary schools since 2011–2012 (Narcotics Division 2017b). The Beat Drugs Fund continued to provide a whale of resources to projects in drug prevention, treatment, as well as research.

The percentage of persons under the age of 21 among all reported persons in CRDA data began to drop in 2011 (see Table 1.2). This may have partly been due to the tremendous efforts made by the government and NGOs in prevention and T&R

work over the past several years. While the prevalence rate of young people's drug use may have dropped, there is evidence that more and more adolescent drug users have become "hidden" (taking drugs at home or friend's home), posting an increasingly serious problem to policy makers and service providers.

Social Change and Young People's Drug Use in Hong Kong

1950s–1980s

Young people are largely products of the society they grow up in. The formation and development of their patterns of attitude and behaviour are inevitably shaped by the social, economic, political, and cultural conditions of the society. In order to gain insights into the recent transition from heroin dominance to the popularity of psychoactive drugs among young people, let us briefly examine the social change that has occurred in Hong Kong since the mid-twentieth century.

When Hong Kong became a British colony in the second half of the nineteenth century, it was only a small fishing village with a sparse population. Hong Kong had always been a haven for scores of people who fled Mainland China during times of natural disasters, civil wars, and China's war against Japanese invasion (1937–1945) in the first half of the twentieth century. But it was not until the late 1940s, when the Communists were about to win the civil war over the Nationalists, that massive inflow of people from the Mainland to Hong Kong did the population of Hong Kong experience a drastic upsurge. Soon after the Communists established their regime on the Mainland in 1949, Mainlanders were not permitted to freely enter Hong Kong.

The large number of new arrivals became a driving force for the economic growth of Hong Kong. While the majority of them were manual labourers, some of them were entrepreneurs in manufacturing and other industries based mainly in the commercial city of Shanghai who closed their businesses to come to Hong Kong before 1949. The availability of cheap labour, capital, and technical know-how, coupled with the government's laissez-faire and free-port policy, had facilitated the development of industrialization in the 1960s. Being a busy entrepot, as well as an export-oriented economy supported by the proliferation of small factories, Hong Kong quickly became a successful export-processing zone (King and Man 1979; Leung 1996). By the 1980s, Hong Kong had become one of the "Four Little Dragons" in East Asia (Hong Kong, Taiwan, South Korea, and Singapore) as well as one of the largest financial centres in the world. Fast industrialization and economic growth had resulted in greater educational opportunities for the younger generation, including university education, expansion of the job market, and rise of the standard of living. The middle class had greatly expanded; and upward mobility was not a far-fledged dream any more for many ambitious lower-class people. In a way, that was a time that the "Hong Kong Dream" could come true.

During the period of fast economic growth as well as increasing industrialization and modernization from the 1960s to 1980s, the prevalence of drug abuse in young people had been low (see figures for the selected years of the 1980s in Table 1.2). The increase of opportunities for upward mobility in this period was definitely a protective factor against drug abuse in young people, but there were at least two other favourable factors. First, groundwork for a more comprehensive approach to drug work of the government and NGOs had been laid during the period of 1960s–1980s. In response to the high prevalence of heroin addiction in the 1950s, the government and the public began to initiate treatment facilities for addicts. Since the 1960s, besides implementing mandatory treatment to prison inmates with known drug addictions, voluntary treatment programmes were also set up. In addition, a voluntary outpatient methadone treatment programme was experimented in 1972, and then full fledgedly set up in 1976, for heroin treatment and maintenance purposes. While there was fast expansion of the quantity and variety of treatment services, drug prevention gradually became a new area of drug work. Since the 1980s, prevention efforts in the form of school talks and exhibition as well as public education through posters, TV and other media announcements, and community prevention activities were promoted by both the government and NGOs. The trend of drug abuse of adults and adolescents was monitored by CRDA mentioned above and the conducting of school surveys once every 2 or 3 years. Although Hong Kong's drug policy, like those of many countries, basically adopts a prohibition framework, the incorporation and proliferation of treatment and prevention strategies in the three decades between 1960s and 1980s can be described as a period of what the senior author has called "Enlightened Prohibition" (Cheung and Ch'ien 1996). A drug policy that emphasized treatment and prevention besides law enforcement must have contributed to the relatively low prevalence of drug abuse among young people in those days.

Another possible reason for the low levels of drug abuse in young people between 1960s and 1980s was a sociocultural one. While the 1960s marked the beginning of rapid industrialization and modernization, Hong Kong was still predominantly a Chinese society in terms of population and culture (Chan and Lee 1995). In traditional Chinese culture, the family is the most important functioning social and economic unit, whose members put the family's interest and well-being before theirs. Authority is distributed hierarchically according to age and gender. Since the 1950s, the importance of the family was further reinforced by the "refugee mentality" in the majority of the population in Hong Kong who were migrants from the Mainland. As "refugees" from China, they were relieved to be able to flee from the Mainland and thus would not expect the colonial government in Hong Kong to provide them with much social welfare and service. They relied on their own families as sources of livelihood and welfare. Individual members of the family worked hard for the benefit of the whole family. This practical aspect of the family in Hong Kong was described by Lau as "utilitarianistic familism" (Lau 1981). In such a traditional and materialistic Chinese family, parenting tended to be strict and repressive (Lin and Fu 1990; Wu 1996), and obedience of children was taken for granted, in contrast to the lack of emphasis placed on independence, assertiveness, and creativity (Ho

1986). The informal control of the family over its children was tight. Physical punishment was widely practised (Leung and Fan 1996). Chinese parents' controlling pattern did not necessarily imply domination but involved organizational pattern of control which shows high support and investment of input in children's development (McBride-Chang and Chang 1998). It follows that children accepted such parental control, perceiving it as an expression of parental warmth (Chao 1994). Similarly, the school was also a place where students were subject to strict discipline and control. Being the most fundamental socialization and informal social control agents, the family and school must have been very strong protective factors against teenage and adolescent involvement in drug abuse as well as other forms of delinquency in the period of 1950s–1980s (Leung and Fan 1996).

1990s–2010s

We have pointed out above that there occurred a rather sudden sharp turn upwards in the prevalence of drug use in young people as well as the replacement of heroin by psychoactive drugs such as ketamine since 2000 (Table 1.2). Why did these changes happen? We have explored two possible social factors that had helped to protect young people from involvement in drug abuse in 1950s–1980s: (1) expansion of educational and job opportunities due to fast economic growth and (2) the strict informal control of the family and school. Could it be that these two factors have changed, so that their protective effects have diminished since the 1990s? We think so. Let us discuss each of these two societal factors below.

Since Mainland China implemented its economic reform policy around 1980, many owners of manufacturing industries in Hong Kong had gradually moved their factories to South China because labour and infrastructure there were much cheaper than in Hong Kong. By the 1990s, only a minority of factories had remained in Hong Kong, and the once industry-based economy had gradually transformed into a financial one, heavily dependent on the stock and property markets, offering opportunities for quick returns of financial investments and speculations. The Gini coefficient showing the gap between the rich and the poor has risen sharply, from 0.476 in 1991 to 0.518 in 1996, 0.525 in 2001, 0.533 in 2006, 0.537 in 2011, and 0.539 in 2016 (Census and Statistics Department 2001, 2016). In education, although free primary and junior secondary school education has been implemented by the government since 1970, and free senior secondary school education since 2008, and although the number of publicly funded universities has increased from two in the 1960s to ten nowadays, entrance into universities remains very competitive (around 38% of young people can receive higher education, subsidized and private, at a degree level) (Legislative Council Panel on Education 2014). For the majority of young people, upward mobility is a very far-fletched dream. A more recent research attempt to gauge the altered nature of the school-to-work transition in Hong Kong is Wu's (2010) longitudinal cohort analysis. Precarious transitions from school to work are found to be more pronounced in the post-1980s young cohort (who were 18–22 years at the time of interview) than in the earlier 1950s, 1960s, and 1970s generations. For the "post-1980" generation of young people, college degrees no longer ensure managerial/professional occupations, and they are increasingly driven to associate professional/clerical occupations and, to some extent, service/sales jobs. Those with associate degrees or other sub-degrees or below are left with lower-level occupations. Whereas there is no decline in the intergenerational upward mobility over cohorts, the intragenerational upward mobility to middle-class status is shrinking for the post-1980s cohort.

While structural changes in the economy since the 1980s had begun to restrict the upward mobility of young people, the protective functions of the family and school against drug abuse and other delinquent behaviours in adolescents had also weakened. Children born in the 1980s in Hong Kong, like their counterparts in many countries, grew up in a globalized and materialistic society where the values of consumerism, individualism, and personal pursuit of success prevail (Chiu 2005; Kam and Harrison 2001). They were not ready to be unconditionally obedient and submissive to their parents or other authorities (Yau and Smetana 2003). This was coupled with the increasing use of a more liberal and humanistic approach to parenting and schooling as a characteristic of modernization. Repressive measures in the family and school such as physical punishment gradually gave way to more child- and student-oriented methods. While such a humanistic shift was socially progressive, the role of parents and teachers in value transmission and informal control was inevitably diminished and become less effective (Kam and Harrison 2001).

One way to make sense of the weakening of informal social control functions of the family, school, and other social institutions in society is to borrow the insights of Beck's "risk society" perspective (Beck 1992) in order to understand the social change that has occurred in Hong Kong in the past two decades. A feature of social development in the post-industrialization period is the emergence of the stage of "reflexive modernization", at which a great variety of risks, natural and man-made, are so abundant in society that existing social structures and institutions are increasingly unable to predict and prevent them. A process of individualization gradually occurs, as the individual (agency) is relying less and less on existing social institutions (structure) to predict and handle risks, thereby becoming more and more dissociated from them. Faced with uncertainties and insecurities, individuals have to calculate risks and make decisions for themselves accordingly.

The idea of risk society was nicely applied by the British sociologist, Howard Parker, in explaining the upsurge of drug use in young people nowadays (Parker et al. 1998; Aldridge et al. 2011). Growing up in a risk society, and much more dissociated from conventional institutions such as the family and school than their counterparts in the past, young people today have to get used to understanding and assessing the risks by themselves in everyday life. However, the society is becoming increasingly complicated and changing more and more quickly. As if this is not bad enough, tough competition in society brings more uncertainties and anxieties for young people as they function and adapt daily in a range of roles, contexts, situations, familial, social and community networks, and organizational systems. It is now very difficult for them to perform accurate risk calculation and predict the future. Following conventional rules, such as being a good kid and studying hard, could not guarantee success in their future. Against this background, the consumption of drugs in the party setting of heavy music and vigorous dancing can be seen as being a viable, available, and accessible response mechanism to the uncertain and tough reality facing young people. In the temporary escape, they enjoy a moment of stability and security as well as reconstruct their youth identity. Parker designated the increasing popularity of party drug use as "normalization of recreational drug use". Many young people are increasingly receptive to recreational drug use and involved in it. Unlike the previous pattern of young people's drug use in the 1970s and 1980s, when heroin was the dominant drug and heroin abuse was more commonly found in young people in lower socioeconomic conditions, the popularity of party drug use cuts across gender, age, education, and occupation lines.

Parker and his team studied the normalization of recreational drug use in the UK and their thesis has garnered considerable support in a variety of Western contexts (e.g. Bahora et al. 2009; Fitzgerald et al. 2013; Pape and Rossow 2004; Pilkington 2007; van der Poel et al. 2009; Sznitman 2007; Sznitman et al. 2013; Wilson et al. 2010; also see Sznitman and Taubman 2016 for a recent review) and has been used to address racial-ethnic acculturation (Moloney et al. 2008) and integration of urban-rural dichotomies (van Hout 2011). In Hong Kong, we have examined the normalization phenomenon in the mid-2000s (Cheung and Cheung 2006) and concluded that, although not as fully fledged as that in the UK, normalization had indeed occurred in Hong Kong by the mid-2000s, as indicated by young people's growing receptiveness to occasional drug use and the upsurge in the prevalence of psychoactive drug use in them. We also pointed out that the weakening of social structural forces in the family, school, and community might have contributed to the normalization process (Cheung 2015). Young drug users in Hong Kong now do not only exhibit a high degree of permissiveness to recreational drug use, they have also developed a unique method of "neutralization" that has facilitated the normalization process in Hong Kong.

Neutralization of Recreational Drug Use

In the midst of decreasing influence and control from family and school, youngsters develop their own view of benefits and harms of their drugs of choice, and balance the pleasure and harm of drug use. In this context, a new drug use subculture has occurred in Hong Kong, involving a process of neutralization of psychoactive drug use quite unique to Hong Kong (Cheung 2015). It is a common perception, or misperception, among young people that drugs can be divided into two broad types. Heroin and other drugs in the narcotics category are "hard drugs", whereas psychoactive drugs such as ketamine, ecstasy, ice, and cannabis are "soft drugs". Many young drug users think that, as soft drugs, psychoactive drugs are not as scary as heroin. It is not as easy to get addicted to as is heroin, and even if one becomes addicted, it is easier to quit. The harm of soft drugs, such as ketamine, is perceived by young drug users as not serious (Joe Laidler 2005). Contrarily, heroin is perceived as being much more dangerous. It is easy to get addicted to, and difficult to quit, and the physical harm is much greater than ketamine. This comparison has created the myth that as long as they don't "do heroin", they are safe. Regarding method of administration, ketamine is very easy to use – simply by snorting. Snorting ketamine powder at home, on the street, or even in school or workplace would not be easily noticed. In addition, in the eyes of young people, heroin represents an outdated drug popular among the older generation, but ketamine is trendy. When consumed in a party setting, ketamine produces a spiritual awakening and liberation (Joe Laidler and Hunt 2013). In young people's risk calculation, the pleasure of ketamine use far outweighs its harm.

In addition to comparing psychoactive drugs with heroin with regard to addictiveness, bodily harm, and trendiness, the use of ketamine and other psychoactive drugs was also defined in such a way that fostered the neutralization process. Ketamine use was considered as being a "bad habit" rather than drug abuse. Many young people have a variety of bad habits, ranging from smoking, drinking, gambling to gang fighting, skipping school, and premarital sex. Snorting ketamine is no more than one of the common bad habits in many youngsters. Bad habits are not good but are not a big deal either. They are not something that belong exclusively to unruly adolescents. Those so-called good students also have bad habits; and even parents and teachers have bad habits. The reduction of "drug abuse" to "bad habit", or what we have called *bad habitization* of drug use (Cheung and Zhong 2014), is a way to neutralize the behaviour of psychoactive drug abuse. It brings negative consequences such as lowering the awareness of the danger of psychoactive drug abuse, encouraging the denial of drug abuse, and undermining the motivation to seek help.

Summary

This chapter has briefly reviewed the major changes of the drug scene in Hong Kong since the mid-1990s, namely, (i) the upsurge of the use of psychoactive drugs, especially ketamine, among young people and (ii) the replacement of heroin by ketamine as the drug of choice among young drug users. Social change that has occurred in Hong Kong since the 1950s may provide some clues to the understanding of the rapidly growing drug use among young people since the 1990s. Hong Kong had experienced a process of rapid industrialization and modernization in the 1960s and 1970s, boosting the economy and increasing the availability of upward mobility for young people. This could have increased their stake of conformity and reduced their likelihood of engaging in deviant behaviour. The Chinese traditional culture of submission to the authority and control of the family and school was still effectively preventing young people from deviating excessively from social norms. Things began to change in the 1980s, when Mainland China's economic reform quickly resulted in the restructuring of the Hong Kong economy from an industrial economy to financial-based economy in which speculations in the stock and property market were rampant. The gap between the rich and the poor was quickly widening, and the opportunities for young people to achieve upward mobility were becoming stringent. At the same time, the traditional informal social control functions of social institutions such as the family and school were challenged by the younger generation, who were increasingly dissociated from conventional social structural constraints and making decisions for themselves in the highly competitive world. A coping mechanism for uncertainties and insecurities was to engage in parties or social gatherings, where recreational drug use was an integral part. Moreover, the neutralization of ketamine and other psychoactive drug use, involving a comparison of ketamine with heroin in addictiveness, bodily harm, and trendiness, and the definition of ketamine use as bad habit rather than drug abuse, has facilitated the process of recreational drug use in Hong Kong.

References

Aldridge, J., Measham, F., & Willams, L. (2011). *Illegal leisure revisited: Changing patterns of alcohol and drug use in adolescents and young adults*. New York: Routledge.

Bahora, M., Sterk, C. E., & Elifson, K. W. (2009). Understanding recreational ecstasy use in the United States: A qualitative inquiry. *International Journal of Drug Policy, 20*, 62–69.

Beck, U. (1992). *Risk society: Towards a new modernity*. London: Sage.

Census and Statistics Department. (2001). *2001 population census: Summary results*. Hong Kong: Census and Statistics Department.

Census and Statistics Department. (2016). 2016 population by-census. In*Thematic report: Household income distribution in Hong Kong*. Hong Kong: Census and Statistics Department.

Chan, H. M., & Lee, R. P. L. (1995). Hong Kong families: At the crossroads of modernism and traditionalism. *Journal of Comparative Family Studies, 26*, 83–99.

Chao, R. K. (1994). Beyond parental control and authoritarian parenting style: Understanding Chinese parenting through the cultural notion of training. *Child Development, 65*, 1111–1120.

Cheung, Y. W. (1998). The hidden challenges. *Spotlight, 28*, 7–9. November (Published by the Hong Kong Council of Social Service).

Cheung, Y. W. (2000). Substance abuse and developments in harm reduction. *Canadian Medical Association Journal, 162*(12), 1697–1700.

Cheung, Y. W. (2015). Macro social flaws and intervention's unfinished business: A personal note on young people's drug use in Hong Kong. *Substance Use & Misuse, 50*, 1044–1050.

Cheung, Y. W., & Ch'ien, J. M. N. (1996). Drug use and drug policy in Hong Kong: Changing patterns and new challenges. *Substance Use & Misuse, 31*(11 & 12), 1573–1597.

Cheung, N. W. T., & Cheung, Y. W. (2006). Is Hong Kong experiencing normalization of adolescent drug use? Some reflections on the normalization thesis. *Substance Use & Misuse, 41*(14), 1967–1990.

Cheung, Y. W., & Zhong, S. H. (2014). Official reactions to crime and drug problems in Hong Kong. In C. Liqun, I. Sun, & B. Hebenton (Eds.), *The Routledge handbook of Chinese criminology* (pp. 295–308). Oxon: Routledge.

Chiu, S. W. S. (2005). Rethinking youth problem in a risk society: Some reflections on working with 'youth-at-risk' in Hong Kong. In F. W. L. Lee (Ed.), *Working with youth-at-risk in Hong Kong* (pp. 99–112). Hong Kong: Hong Kong University Press.

Fitzgerald, R., Mazerolle, L., & Mazerolle, P. (2013). Drug normalization and Australian youth: Group differences in the social accommodation of drug use. *Journal of Youth Studies, 16*, 901–915.

Ho, D. Y. F. (1986). Chinese patterns of socialization: A critical review. In M. H. Bond (Ed.), *The psychology of the Chinese people* (pp. 1–35). Hong Kong: Oxford University Press.

van Hout, M. C. (2011). Differentiated normalization and drug transitions among rural youth in Ireland. *Drugs: Education, Prevention and Policy, 18*, 124–131.

Hsü, I. C. Y. (1995). *The rise of modern China* (5th ed.). New York: Oxford University Press.

Joe Laidler, K. A. (2005). The rise of club drugs in a heroin society: The case of Hong Kong. *Substance Use & Misuse, 40*, 1257–1278.

Joe Laidler, K. A., & Hunt, G. (2013). Unlocking the spiritual with club drugs: A case study of two youth cultures. *Substance Use & Misuse, 48*, 1099–1108.

Kam, Y. M., & Harrison, L. (2001). Globalisation, cultural change and the modern drug epidemics: The case of Hong Kong. *Health, Risk & Society, 3*, 39–57.

King, A. Y. C., & Man, P. J. L. (1979). Small factory in economic development: The case of Hong Kong. In T. B. Lin, R. P. L. Lee, & U. E. Simons (Eds.), *Hong Kong: Economic, social and political studies in development* (pp. 31–63). White Plains: M.E. Sharpe.

Lau, S. K. (1981). Utilitarianistic familism: The basis of political stability. In A. Y. V. King & R. P. L. Lee (Eds.), *Social life and development in Hong Kong* (pp. 195–216). Hong Kong: The Chinese University Press.

Legislative Council Panel on Education. (2014). *Discussion paper on enhancing the transparency and quality of the self-financing post-secondary sector*. Hong Kong: Legislative Council.

Leung, B. K. P. (1996). *Perspectives on Hong Kong society*. Hong Kong: Oxford University Press.

Leung, K., & Fan, R. M. T. (1996). Adolescent delinquent behavior in Chinese societies. In S. Lau (Ed.), *Growing up the Chinese way: Chinese child and adolescent development* (pp. 237–264). Hong Kong: The Chinese University Press.

Lin, C. C. Y., & Fu, V. R. (1990). A comparison of child-rearing practices among Chinese, immigrant Chinese, and Caucasian-American parents. *Child Development, 61*, 429–433.

McBride-Chang, C., & Chang, L. (1998). Adolescent-parent relations in Hong Kong: Parenting styles, emotional autonomy, and school achievement. *The Journal of Genetic Psychology: Research and Theory on Human Development, 159*, 421–436.

Moloney, M., Hunt, G., & Evans, K. (2008). Asian American identity and drug consumption: From acculturation to normalization. *Journal of Ethnicity in Substance Abuse, 7*, 376–403.

Narcotics Division. (1982). *Central registry of drug abuse ninth report (September 1976 – December 1881)*. Hong Kong: Narcotics Division, Security Bureau, Government of Hong Kong.

Narcotics Division. (2011). *Evaluation research of trial scheme on school drug tests in Tai Po District (school year 2010/11)*. Hong Kong: Narcotics Division, Security Bureau, Government of the Hong Kong SAR.

Narcotics Division. (2014). *Central registry of drug abuse sixty-third report (2004–2013)*. Hong Kong: Narcotics Division, Security Bureau, Government of the Hong Kong SAR.

Narcotics Division. (2017a). *Beat drugs fund*. Hong Kong: Narcotics Division, Security Bureau, Government of the Hong Kong SAR. In website of Narcotics Division: http://www.nd.gov.hk/en/beat.htm. Access date: April 9, 2017.

Narcotics Division. (2017b). *Healthy school programme*. Hong Kong: Narcotics Division, Security Bureau, Government of the Hong Kong SAR. In website of Narcotics Division: http://www.nd.gov.hk/en/HSP.htm. Access date: April 9, 2017.

Pape, H., & Rossow, I. (2004). 'Ordinary' people with 'normal' lives? A longitudinal study of ecstasy and other drug use among Norwegian youth. *Journal of Drug Issues, 34*, 389–418.

Parker, H., Aldridge, J., & Measham, F. (1998). *Illegal leisure: The normalization of adolescent recreational drug use*. London: Routledge.

Pilkington, H. (2007). Beyond 'peer pressure': Rethinking drug use and 'youth culture'. *International Journal of Drug Policy, 18*, 213–224.

van der Poel, A., Rodenburg, G., Dijkstra, M., Stoele, M., & van de Mheen, D. (2009). Trends, motivations and settings of recreational cocaine use by adolescents and young adults in the Netherland. *International Journal of Drug Policy, 20*, 143–151.

Sznitman, S. R. (2007). An examination of the normalization of cannabis use among 9th grade school students in Sweden and Switzerland. *Addiction Research and Theory, 15*, 601–616.

Sznitman, S. R., & Taubman, D. S. (2016). Drug use normalization: A systematic and critical mixed-methods review. *Journal of Studies in Alcohol and Drugs, 77*, 700–709.

Sznitman, S. R., Kolobov, T., der Bogt, T., Kuntsche, E., Walsh, S. D., Boniel-Nissim, M., & Harel-Fisch, Y. (2013). Exploring substance abuse normalization among adolescents: A multilevel study of 35 countries. *Social Science & Medicine, 97*, 143–151.

Task Force on Youth Drug Abuse. (2008). *Report of the task force on youth drug abuse*. Hong Kong: Government of the Hong Kong SAR.

Traver, H. H. (1992). Colonial relations and opium control policy in Hong Kong, 1841–1945. In H. H. Traver & M. G. Gaylord (Eds.), *Drugs, law and the state* (pp. 135–149). Hong Kong: Hong Kong University Press.

Wilson, H., Bryant, J., Holt, M., & Treloar, C. (2010). Normalisation of recreational drug use among young people: Evidence about accessibility, use and contact with other drug users. *Health Sociology Review, 19*, 164–175.

Wu, D. Y. H. (1996). Parental control: Psychocultural interpretation of Chinese patterns of socialization. In S. Lau (Ed.), *Growing up the Chinese way: Chinese child and adolescent development* (pp. 1–28). Hong Kong: The Chinese University Press.

Wu, X. (2010). *Hong Kong's post-80s generation: Profiles and predicaments, A report commissioned by the Central Policy Unit*. China: Government of the Hong Kong SAR.

Yau, J., & Smetana, J. (2003). Adolescent-parent conflict in Hong Kong and Shenzhen: A comparison of youth in two cultural contexts. *International Journal of Behavioral Development, 27*, 201–211.

Chapter 2
A Longitudinal Survey of Psychoactive Drug Abusers in Hong Kong

When ketamine first appeared in CRDA's record in 2000 and then quickly became a dominant psychoactive drug among young people (Table 1.2), youth workers, health professionals, parents, teachers, and government officials were caught by surprise. Very little was known about the drug and its abusers. The serious lack of knowledge of the drug had made medical treatment of ketamine abuse and prevention work in young people difficult. Since the mid-2000s, there has been a large amount of clinical research conducted to find out the physical harms and mental impairment of ketamine abuse (e.g. Chan 2012; Chan et al. 2013; Liang et al. 2013, 2014; Poon et al. 2010; Tam et al. 2016; Tang et al. 2013; Wang et al. 2013; Wei et al. 2013; Wong et al. 2014; Yew 2015). The availability of medical research findings on the adverse physical and mental consequences of ketamine abuse has facilitated drug treatment services for ketamine abusers as well as primary and secondary prevention work among young people. By the late 2000s, many ketamine abusers, who started using the drug in the early 2000s, were already in their mid to late 20s having a history of ketamine use for 8 years or more. Such a period was long enough to develop symptoms of serious health problems with the lung, kidney, urinary tract system and bladder, etc. as well as psychosis and other mental impairments. They became vivid and effective examples of victims of ketamine abuse in prevention work among young people.

Equally lacking in the 2000s was the knowledge about ketamine abusers. As the number of young people using ketamine increased quickly since the early 2000s, there was an urgent need to understand what social, demographic, and psychological factors might affect the continuation or discontinuation of drug use among psychoactive drug users. Such research findings would serve as important references for the design of intervention strategies for ketamine addicts. This research gap was partly bridged by a 3-year longitudinal study entitled "A Longitudinal Survey of Psychoactive Drug Abusers in Hong Kong" conducted by the senior author between 2009 and 2011, with funding from the Beat Drugs Fund of the government (Cheung 2012).

Y.W. Cheung, N.W.-t. Cheung, *Psychoactive Drug Abuse in Hong Kong*,
Quality of Life in Asia 11, DOI 10.1007/978-981-10-6154-7_2

The major objective of the longitudinal study was to find the socio-demographic and psychosocial factors that might be conducive to the continuation or discontinuation of drug use of a group of identified psychoactive drug abusers (the other two objectives were to study the harmful effects of psychoactive abuse reported by the subjects and to assess the economic cost of psychoactive drug abuse in society). This book reports the results of a detailed analysis of socio-demographic and psychosocial factors affecting drug use of the sample of the longitudinal study.

The Study and Method

A total of 36 youth outreach and treatment and rehabilitation agencies participated in the longitudinal study (Cheung 2012:5–6). Subjects were recruited from the clients of these agencies. The criterion for selection was "have ever used a psychoactive drug". As mentioned in the previous chapter, the definition of "psychoactive drug" used in the study followed the categorization used by the Narcotics Division, Security Bureau, which broadly divided substance of abuse into "narcotics analgesics" and "psychotropic substances". The former includes heroin, opium, morphine, and physeptone/methadone, and the latter includes hallucinogens, depressants, stimulants, tranquillizers, and other substances such as ketamine, cough medicine, and organic solvents (Narcotics Division 2014). The term "psychoactive drug" used in this study was the same as "psychotropic drug" used by the Narcotics Division.

Most clients of the agencies were users of one or more psychoactive drugs. We knew that among psychoactive drug users, ketamine has been the dominant drug, although a wide range of other psychoactive drugs were also consumed. In fact, the boundary between ketamine and other psychoactive drugs was always crossed, due to the popularity of multiple psychoactive drug use.

Altogether, those 36 participating agencies recruited a total of 754 subjects for the baseline T1 sample. The panel of subjects were interviewed six times, spaced out at 6-month intervals, so that altogether six waves of interviews were conducted. Most of the agencies were able to arrange for social workers to conduct the interviews. Each agency assigned a staff member to be the coordinator of the team of interviewers. He/she was responsible for maintaining the master list of subjects, distributing questionnaires to interviewers and collecting from them after completion, keeping records of all the subjects, and arranging for interviews at the appropriate time points. He/she also served as the contact person for the Research Assistant of the survey research team at The Chinese University of Hong Kong. In addition to interviewing subjects, the staff of the agencies would also keep track of those subjects who had left the agencies or had half disappeared. A small number of the participating agencies were not able to provide any staff to be interviewers. Subjects of these agencies were interviewed by trained interviewers of a private research organization.

There were both advantages and disadvantages with using social worker staff of agencies as interviewers. The first disadvantage was that social workers were not

Table 2.1 The sample from T1 to T6

	T1	T2	T3	T4	T5	T6
No. of subjects from outreach agencies	569	492	377	355	327	276
No. of subjects from residential T&R agencies	185	108	57	21	20	12
Total no. of subjects	754	600	434	376	347	288
Retention rate compared with previous time point (%)	–	79.6	72.3	86.6	92.3	83.0
Retention rate compared with T1 (%)	–	79.6	57.6	49.9	46.0	38.2

professional interviewers. This disadvantage was reduced by organizing briefing sessions on the questionnaire and the interview for the interviewer staff. Their interviewing skills would also improve after the first interview. The second disadvantage was the agency staff's close relationships with their clients. The interview might be affected by how the social worker interviewer evaluated the specific clients being interviewed and vice versa. There might also be the issue of social desirability. A client might under-report his/her drug use or pose a less permissive attitude towards drug use, so as to impress the social worker interviewer in charge of his/her case. To minimize this disadvantage, interviewers were reminded to be as objective as possible during the interview and to motivate their interviewees to be honest in answering questions.

Despite these disadvantages, there were several advantages. Most social workers were able to gain the trust of their clients and establish good rapport with them. This offered a good opportunity for the interview to be successfully conducted. In front of the social worker, who knew his/her clients very well, the client interviewee did not need to hide his/her drug use. If the interviewer was a stranger, it would be much more difficult to obtain honest answers from the client. Thus, we believe that using the agencies' social workers as interviewers was a good strategy for obtaining reliable data. Also, since the staff interviewers and their client interviewees were in the same agency, it was more convenient for the interviews to take place than having to arrange for an external research team to come and do the interviews.

Agency interviewers were encouraged to contact the research team for comments and advice whenever they had any questions regarding the interviews. Meetings were organized for them to share their interview experience and obstacles before new waves of interviews began.

The sample size for T1, and those of subsequent time points, is reported in Table 2.1.

For the T1 baseline survey, 754 subjects were recruited from the agencies, which was an impressive sample size, given that this required the cooperation of a large number of agencies. A large baseline sample was also necessary due to the expected large attrition rates in the course of time (some might finish receiving service from the agency before the end of the study; others might discontinue the service prematurely). Three-quarters (569) of subjects of this sample were recruited from outreach agencies and one-quarter (185) from residential T&R agencies.

Fig. 2.1 Example of "suitable-for-interview" period

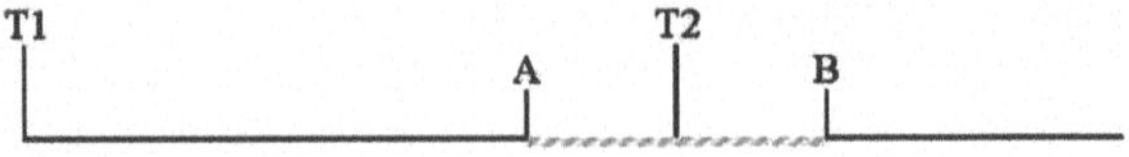

T1 – T2: 6 months between T1 interview and T2 interview
A – T2: 3 weeks before supposed date of T2 interview
T2 – B: 3 weeks after supposed date of T2 interview
A – B: Suitable-for-interview period

From T2 onwards, the number of subjects dropped to 600 at T2, 434 at T3, 376 at T4, 347 at T5, and 288 at T6. The retention rate was 79.6% at T2/T1, 72.3% at T3/T2, 86.6% at T4/T3, 92.3% at T5/T4, and 83.0% at T6/T5. Given that the sample was not a stable one, these retention rates were quite satisfactory. The largest drop-out rates occurred at T2 and T3. Once subjects had been interviewed three times, their continued participation was more easily secured. In fact, we have asked interviewers to issue to each subject a small card upon completion of the T3 interview, noting the dates of interviews for T4, T5, and T6. A small ball pen was also given to each subject as a gift upon finishing the T3 interview. This helped to motivate and remind subjects to participate in the T4 and T5 interviews. As a result, the retention rate was high at T4 and T5, although less satisfactory at T6. If we compare the numbers of subjects from T2 to T6 with reference to the number of subjects at T1, the retention rate decreased from 79.6% at T2 to 57.6% at T3, 49.9% at T4, 46.0% at T5, and 38.2% at T6. A discussion of the drop-out rates at different time points and how they might have affected the overall sample can be found in Appendix One.

In order to increase the incentive of selected agency clients to participate as interviewees of the survey, a remuneration of the amount of HK$100 was rewarded to each subject after successful completion of an interview. Some agencies preferred receiving supermarket coupons of an equivalent amount instead of cash for their client interviewees. Also, as a token gift to agency staff who conducted interviews, an amount of HK$50 was remunerated to the agency for each successful completion of an interview. Some agencies would like to pool together the amounts of remuneration for the subjects and the staff interviewers, in order to use the money to organize activities for their clients.

Consent of the subjects to participate in the six waves of interviews was obtained through consent forms before the first interview. For subjects under the age of 18, parents' consent would be sought. However, many young drug users had poor relationships with their parents, and some of them even ran away from home and did not live with their parents. In such cases, in order not to miss out such cases, social workers would be required to discuss the participation with them and give consent on their behalf. The survey had received approval of the ethics review committee of The Chinese University of Hong Kong.

The six waves of interviews were conducted at 6-month intervals. In principle, the space between two interviews should be 6 months. In reality, some flexibility was necessary, as clients did not always show up at exactly 6-month intervals waiting to be interviewed. We specified a "suitable-for-interview period", in which interviews could be conducted. This period spanned from 3 weeks before the exact 6-month date and 3 weeks after the 6-month date, as shown in Fig. 2.1.

Table 2.2 The five focus groups

Group	No. of participants	Type of participants	Type of agency recruited from	Date
1	7	Male	A youth outreach centre in North District	June 3, 2011
		Age range: 13–17		
		Five attending school		
		Two left school		
2	15	Male	A male residential treatment centre in N.T. West	June 9, 2011
		Age range: 25–30		
3	8	Female	A female residential treatment centre on Hong Kong Island	June 24, 2011
		Age range: 18–30		
4	8	Male	A male residential treatment centre in Kowloon East	July 13, 2011
		Age range: 18–25		
5	5	Female	A female residential treatment centre in Kowloon East	September 6, 2011
		Age range: 20–29		

As some subjects did not show up to their respective agencies regularly, they should be interviewed as soon as they were available, because there was no guarantee that they would make themselves available on the scheduled date of interview later. We set 3 weeks to be the period before the supposed interview date that early interviews could be conducted. For subjects whose agency staff did not get hold of them until after the supposed interview date, there was also a 3-week allowance for the interview to be conducted. Each subject had his/her own "suitable-for-interview" period, and the agency interviewers kept track of their clients' records for interview arrangements.

As agencies did not start their T1 interviews on the same date, the same wave of interviews across agencies spanned about 4 months. The rough dates of the six waves of interviews were as follows:

T1: April–July 2009
T2: October 2009–January 2010
T3: April–July 2010
T4: October 2010–January 2011
T5: April–July 2011
T6: October–December 2011

In addition to the six waves of interviews, five focus group sessions were organized to obtain in-depth qualitative data on a variety of topics such as young people's initiation and progression of drug use, reasons for use, and the adverse effects of psychoactive drug abuse (Table 2.2). Data obtained from focus group sessions were used to interpret the meanings of the quantitative results of the survey. Consent was obtained from each participant before the sessions were conducted. Each focus group member received a remuneration of HK$100 for the participation.

Independent Variables

Socio-demographic Variables

A number of commonly used socio-demographic variables were introduced, including sex, age, number of siblings, marital status, student status (whether a student or not), employment, religion, and housing type.

Psychosocial Variables

A variety of psychosocial variables were used in the study to cover some of the major psychosocial perspectives concerning young people's drug use. They included the following[1]:

Permissiveness to Drug Use

This variable refers to the extent to which drug use is acceptable to the individual. In the above discussion of "normalization of recreational drug use" (Parker et al. 1998), an increasingly permissive attitude towards recreational drug use is one of the elements of normalization. We have also shown that as early as the mid-2000s, a permissive attitude towards drug use was common among marginal youths in Hong Kong (Cheung and Cheung 2006). It is interesting to know whether, among psychoactive drug users themselves, a difference in the level of permisssiveness towards drug use would affect their continuation/discontinuation of drug use.

The variable was formed by four statements: (1) "Abusing drugs is not a proper behaviour (reverse scoring)", (2) "using drugs occasionally is acceptable", (3) "abusing drugs frequently is acceptable", and (4) "abusing drugs when having fun with friends on recreational occasions is okay". Each question was measured by a 4-point scoring system (1=strongly disagree, 2=disagree, 3=agree, 4=strongly agree"). The scale had a score range of 4–16. The alpha value of the scale was .704 at the baseline survey, indicating a high degree of reliability. The higher the degree of permissiveness, the more positive the attitude towards drug use.

---

[1] In the original study, two more psychosocial variables were introduced, namely, "hopelessness" and "having found a goal in life". However, they were not included in this analysis. As a sense of hopelessness was already assessed in Beck's Depression Scale, as well as by the variable "sense of uncertainty about future", the redundancy in assessing hopelessness could be avoided by leaving out the hopelessness variable. As to having found a goal in life, information collected from our focus group sessions with young psychoactive drug users suggested that adolescents were not very clear about what "a goal in life" means, and many of them did not care about finding a goal in life, which was not the same as not having found a goal in life. This confusion in meaning had cast some doubt on the validity of this variable, and thus it was not included.

Apart from being an overall assessment of acceptance of drug use, this variable was also broken down into two components, namely, attitude towards "regular drug use" and attitude towards "occasional drug use". Permissiveness to regular drug use was measured by question (iii) stated above. Permissiveness to occasional drug use was measured by questions (ii) and (iv). The alpha value for permissiveness to occasional use in the baseline sample was 0.76.

Educational Strain

This is a strain experienced by the individual as a result of the discrepancy between his/her aspired educational level and the actual educational level that he/she expects to achieve (or has already achieved, if the subject is not a student anymore). This concept was based on the sociological perspective of anomie theory, which posits that the discrepancy between the aspired goal of economic success in society and the availability of legitimate means to achieve the goal is a source of strain in the individual (Merton 1957). Education is a legitimate and effective path to success in future, and thus it is everyone's wish to be able to achieve a high level of education. Agnew (1992) extended Merton's concept of anomie by including sources of strain other than economic ones, covering any aspect of life. If a strain is not handled properly, anger and other negative emotions would develop, resulting in various kinds of deviant behaviour, including drug abuse. Here, the discrepancy between the aspired level of education and the actual level of education achieved, or expected to achieve, is a source of strain.

Two questions were asked in the questionnaire, one on the aspired education level and the other on how greatly the subject would be disappointed if he/she could not achieve the desired education level in the future. The latter question on the disappointment level, with a 4-point scoring system from 1 (no big deal) to 4 (very disappointed), was used to measure this variable.

Discrimination by Others

Discrimination from other people may create obstacles in the recovery process of active or former addicts. Discrimination may produce a "labelling" effect in active or rehabilitating drug addicts, undermining their self-images and preventing them from changing their addict identity to that of a normal person (Anderson 1993). The stigma itself would produce further drug abuse, encapsulating the addicts in their "addict careers" (Becker 1963; Cheung and Cheung 2003). In this study, the subject was asked whether or not he/she had ever experienced any discrimination from other people (1=never, 2=some, 3=a lot).

Concerning Views of Life

Several questions asked the subjects whether or not they agreed with the following statements about certain aspects of their lives:

- Being satisfied with life.
- Having a sense of uncertainty about future.
- Doing extreme things such as drug use shows vitality of young people.
- Wishing to have own family, job, and normal life in future.
- Thinking that their parents don't know how to teach their children.
- Thinking that their schools don't know how to teach their students.

Having a high level of life satisfaction and wishing to have a family, job, and normal life in future were likely to be protective factors against continuous drug use, whereas having a strong sense of uncertainty about future, believing that doing extreme things shows the vitality of young people, thinking that their parents don't know how to teach children, and thinking that their schools don't know how teach students were likely to be risk factors in continuous drug use. Each of the above items used a 5-point scoring system, with "1" as "strongly disagree", "2" as "disagree", "3" as "no opinion", "4" as "agree", and "5" as "strongly agree".

Self-Esteem

Self-esteem has been shown to be negatively related to substance use and other deviant behaviours, but this finding has not been all that conclusive. Some studies did not find any significant association between low self-esteem and substance use (e.g. Moore et al. 1996; Jones and Heaven 1998).

In this study, Rosenberg's self-esteem scale (Rosenberg 1965) was used to measure the self-esteem of subjects in the sample of psychoactive drug users in the present study. Will a lower self-esteem be conducive to the continuation of drug use in the subjects of this study? The scale consisted of ten questions, each asking the subject to self-evaluate with respect to self-confidence and self-image. A 5-point scoring system was used for the items, and the total score ranged from 5 to 50. The alpha value of the scale was 0.83 in the baseline sample.

Subjective Weathering

This is the feeling of being more "weathered" by tough life compared with other people in the same age group. We developed this concept on the assumption that a life tougher than those of others in the same age group would be a source of relative deprivation and being worn down and hence might be more at risk of committing deviant behaviour as a coping mechanism (Benson 2014). The subjects were asked to compare with people in their similar age cohorts and report whether (1) they feel they are more mature, (2) they had begun to take up household and other duties at a younger age, and (3) they feel older at heart. Each of these three questions had a score range of "1" (less weathered than people in their same age group) to "5" (much more weathered). The alpha value of this scale in the baseline survey was .563, which is of acceptable reliability.

Depression

A simplified version of the Beck Depression Scale (Beck et al. 1961) was used to measure the depression level of the subjects. The simplified version asked the subject if he/she feels sad, feels discouraged about the future, has a hard time enjoying things, feels guilty, is disappointed in himself/herself, blames himself/herself for his/her faults and weaknesses, thinks about killing himself/herself, has no interest in people, puts off making decisions, worries about his/her looks, has to push himself/herself to do things, feels tired, and has no appetite. The Chinese version of the simplified scale had been validated in Hong Kong, and an example of the use of the validated Chinese version is a study of secondary school students in Hong Kong conducted by Mok et al. (2008). The alpha value of the Depression Scale was .850 in the baseline survey sample, indicating a high level of reliability.

Stricken by Stressful Events

The subjects were asked if they had been stricken by any drastic or stressful events in the past 6 months, such as the divorce of parents and loss of a family member. This is one of Agnew's (1992) three types of strain, generated by "exposure to negative stimuli". The experience of traumatic events might result in sorrow and pain for an extended period of time, putting the individual at risk of deviant behaviour such as drug abuse.

Drug Use History Variable

Besides the above-mentioned psychosocial variables, the subject's number of years of drug use was also included as an independent variable. The longer the history of drug use, the more likely the subject would continue to use drugs.

Dependent Variable

The major dependent variable was "drug use in the last 30 days". Subjects were asked to report whether or not they had used illicit drugs in the period of 30 days before the day of interview. The answers were "yes" or "no". For those who answered "yes", they were further asked what drug(s) they had used. All subjects in the sample had used at least one psychoactive drug. In the questionnaire, frequency of drug use was also asked but not quantity. Thus, it was not possible to combine frequency with quantity to construct a drug use variable that could better establish the level of use. In view of this, and noting that the focus of the study was on the continuation or discontinuation of drug use at the six time points, the "yes/no" dichotomy would serve the purpose of the present analysis.

Since this is a longitudinal study involving six waves of data collection, the dependent variable of drug use in the last 30 days would become an independent variable of all the variables at the next time point. Likewise, all the independent variables at a certain time point would be dependent variables for variables at the previous time point.

Characteristics of the Sample

The socio-demographic characteristics of the sample from T1 to T6 were given in Table 2.3 (Cheung 2012).

In the full sample at T1, two-thirds (65.8%) of the subjects were male, and almost three-quarters (72.7%) were below the age of 21. The mean age was 20.6. Two-thirds (66.1%) had one or two siblings. The majority of the subjects (88.8%) had never been married. Almost two-thirds (63.2%) had received only F3 (Grade 9) or less education, whereas one-third (32.8%) had studied up to F4 or F5. Only 31.1% of the subjects were students, and among them, 23.3% were not regularly attending school. Among those who were not students and who were 16 years of age or older, slightly more than half (53.8%) had a job. Only one-third (32%) of the subjects reported having a religion. About one-third (34.7%) of the subjects lived in private housing; others mostly lived in public housing or rooms/quarters. Three subjects were homeless at T1.

In sum, the sample was a young group of psychoactive drug users, mostly male and unmarried, with lower to upper secondary school education, and living in public housing. This fits the social image of young psychoactive drug users in the 2000s.

The turnover of clients in the participating agencies was understandably high. This had posed an obstacle to the interviews. Some subjects finished receiving service from their agencies and left after the first or second interviews. Although agency staff had made tremendous efforts to continue to track these departed subjects down and motivate them to continue with subsequent interviews, some of them would not agree to continue their participation, and others might not be located by former social workers any more. Some interviewees had left their respective agencies prematurely and thus were not to be found. As a result, the sample consisted of unstable subjects, and the drop-out rate was bound to be high (see Table 2.1). Quite expectedly, the drop-out rate was higher among young and male subjects than female and older subjects, as can be seen from Table 2.3.

We next examine the psychosocial characteristics of the sample (Cheung 2012) which were given in Table 2.4.

Table 2.3 Socio-demographic characteristics of the sample

Socio-demographic characteristics	T1		T2		T3		T4		T5		T6	
	%	N	%	N	%	N	%	N	%	N	%	N
Gender		754		600		434		376		347		288
M	65.8	496	63.8	383	63.6	276	60.1	226	61.1	212	58.0	167
F	34.2	258	36.2	217	36.4	158	39.9	150	38.9	135	42.0	121
Age	$(\bar{x} = 20.6; N = 754)$		$(\bar{x} = 20.3; N = 600)$		$(\bar{x} = 20.2; N = 434)$		$(\bar{x} = 19.8; N = 360)$		$(\bar{x} = 20.5; N = 346)$		$(\bar{x} = 20.7; N = 288)$	
12–16	32.2	243	28.7	172	23.0	100	16.5	47	8.1	28	5.9	17
17–20	40.5	305	45.5	273	50.7	220	56.8	213	58.4	202	54.2	156
21–30	16.9	128	17.7	106	19.6	85	23.2	87	29.2	101	36.8	106
31 or over	10.3	78	8.2	49	3.8	29	3.5	13	4.3	15	3.1	9
No. of siblings		742		590		429		374		343		284
0	12.7	94	13.1	77	13.1	56	9.9	37	10.2	35	12.3	35
1–2	66.1	500	68.1	402	69.5	298	72.7	272	72.3	248	71.1	202
3 or more	21.2	148	18.8	111	17.5	75	17.4	65	17.5	60	16.5	47
Marital status		752		600		431		276		347		288
Never married	88.8	668	91.5	549	86.6	376	83.8	315	79.5	276	77.1	222
Married	11.2	84	8.4	51	13.3	58	10.9	61	20.5	71	22.9	66
Education		753		598		434		376		347		287
Primary	5.4	41	3.8	23	3.5	15	2.1	8	1.7	6	1.4	4
F1–F3	57.8	436	58.1	347	53.0	230	51.1	192	49.2	171	45.6	131
F4–F5	32.8	247	34.6	207	38.9	169	41.5	156	42.1	146	44.9	129
Beyond F5	4.0	30	3.6	21	4.7	20	5.3	20	6.9	24	8.0	23
Whether still a student		753		600		434		376		346		287
Yes, always attending school	23.1	174	22.2	133	21.2	92	17.6	66	15.0	51	13.2	38

(continued)

Table 2.3 (continued)

Socio-demographic characteristics	T1		T2		T3		T4		T5		T6	
	%	N	%	N	%	N	%	N	%	N	%	N
Yes, but not always attending	7.0	53	6.8	41	9.2	40	2.2	17	5.0	18	3.1	9
No	69.9	526	71.0	426	69.6	302	77.9	293	80.0	277	83.6	240
Employment (non-student and ≥16)		478		398		287		285		273		235
No	46.2	221	49.0	195	41.0	119	36.1	103	32.2	88	34.0	80
Yes	53.8	257	51.0	203	59.0	168	63.9	182	67.8	185	66.0	155
Religion		752		598		434		376		347		288
No	68.0	511	67.7	405	70.0	304	74.5	280	74.1	257	69.4	200
Christianity/Catholicism	24.8	186	25.2	151	24.4	106	18.7	70	19.8	69	23.6	68
Buddhism-Taoism/other	7.2	55	7.1	42	5.5	24	6.9	26	6.1	21	6.9	20
Housing type		754		597		434		376		347		288
Public (rental or self-owned)	58.8	443	60.7	362	60.6	263	62.5	235	60.8	211	59.0	170
Private (rental or self-owned)	34.7	262	34.4	205	33.4	145	31.9	120	32.9	114	35.1	101
Room, quarters, other	6.1	46	4.7	28	6.0	26	5.3	20	6.4	22	5.9	17
Homeless	0.4	3	0.3	2	0.0	0	0.3	1	0.0	0	0.0	0

Table 2.4 Psychosocial characteristics of the sample

Psychosocial characteristics	T1 (N varies from 542 to 587) x̄ (s.d.)	T2 (N varies from 446 to 497) x̄ (s.d.)	T3 (N varies from 345 to 377) x̄ (s.d.)	T4 (N varies from 326 to 357) x̄ (s.d.)	T5 (N varies from 285 to 327) x̄ (s.d.)	T6 (N varies from 245 to 277) x̄ (s.d.
No. of years of drug use	3.40	3.83	4.39	5.08	5.64	6.19
	(3.14)	(3.21)	(3.16)	(3.76)	(3.68)	(3.45)
Permissiveness to drug use	9.26	8.87	8.64	8.24	8.08	8.06
(4 = lowest; 16 = highest)	(2.19)	(2.29)	(2.22)	(2.19)	(2.37)	(2.41)
How disappointed if aspired education level not achieved	2.25	2.22	2.11	2.11	2.10	2.03
(1 = not disappointed, 4 = v. disappointed)	(1.11)	(1.04)	(1.02)	(1.06)	(0.99)	(1.00)
Ever been discriminated by other people	1.41	1.29	1.26	1.25	1.26	1.26
(1 = no; 3 = a lot)	(0.56)	(0.50)	(0.48)	(0.46)	(0.48)	(0.47)
Satisfied with life	3.01	3.18	3.21	3.27	3.38	3.40
(1 = strongly disagree; 5 = strongly agree)	(1.04)	(1.03)	(1.05)	(1.06)	(1.05)	(0.96)
Sense of uncertainty about future	3.81	3.66	3.68	3.56	3.46	3.46
(1 = strongly disagree; 5 = strongly agree)	(0.87)	(0.90)	(0.91)	(0.90)	(0.87)	(0.87)
Thought doing extreme things shows vitality of your people	2.64	2.45	2.35	2.29	2.29	2.23
(1 = strongly disagree; 5 = strongly agree)	(1.07)	(0.98)	(0.92)	(1.01)	(0.99)	(0.99)
Wish to have own family, job, and normal life in future	4.39	4.29	4.37	4.41	4.34	4.22
(1 = strongly disagree: 5 = strongly agree)	(0.71)	(0.71)	(0.71)	(0.73)	(0.72)	(0.79)

(continued)

Table 2.4 (continued)

Psychosocial characteristics	T1 (N varies from 542 to 587) x̄ (s.d.)	T2 (N varies from 446 to 497) x̄ (s.d.)	T3 (N varies from 345 to 377) x̄ (s.d.)	T4 (N varies from 326 to 357) x̄ (s.d.)	T5 (N varies from 285 to 327) x̄ (s.d.)	T6 (N varies from 245 to 277) x̄ (s.d.
Thought own parents didn't know how to teach children	2.83	2.82	2.78	2.69	2.69	2.72
(1 = strongly disagree; 5 = strongly agree)	(1.14)	(1.11)	(1.10)	(1.15)	(1.09)	(1.01)
Thought own school didn't know how to teach students	3.28	3.20	3.23	3.08	3.04	3.05
(1 = strongly disagree; 5 = strongly agree)	(1.15)	(1.13)	(1.15)	(1.15)	(1.11)	(1.13)
Self-esteem	31.76	32.63	33.44	33.79	34.10	34.40
(10 = lowest; 50 = highest)	(6.19)	(5.89)	(5.66)	(5.56)	(5.35)	(5.67)
Subjective maturity compared with same age group	8.38	8.37	7.95	7.84	7.83	7.87
(3 = much more mature; 15 = much less mature)	(2.14)	(2.23)	(2.16)	(2.14)	(2.15)	(2.18)
Depression	13.43	13.17	13.13	13.17	13.06	13.07
(0 = lowest; 39 = highest)	(1.45)	(0.94)	(0.55)	(1.08)	(0.42)	(0.48)
Stricken by drastic events in last 6 months	1.44	1.41	1.30	1.24	1.23	1.18
(1 = no; 2 = yes)	(0.49)	(0.46)	(0.46)	(0.43)	(0.42)	(0.39)
Drug use in last 30 days	1.67	1.49	1.39	1.36	1.28	1.27
(1 = no; 2 = yes)	(0.47)	(0.50)	(0.49)	(0.48)	(0.45)	(0.44)

Let us firstly examine the full sample at T1. Subjects of the sample generally did not have a long history of drug use (average number of years of drug use experience was 3.4). This was due to the fact that a majority of the subjects were young. The mean score of permissiveness to drug use in the subjects was 9.26, which is at the medium level of permissiveness (score ranged from 4 to 16). When asked how disappointed they would be if they knew they could not achieve the level of education they aspired, the subjects either would not be disappointed at all or would just be a little bit disappointed. A majority of subjects either had not experienced discrimination from other people or had only sometimes experienced it. Regarding a list of questions asking about attitudes towards certain aspects of life as well as the family and school (5-point scale for each), the subjects obtained medium scores for "satisfied with life" ($\overline{x}$=3.01), a relatively higher score for "sense of uncertainty about future" ($\overline{x}$=3.81), and a relatively low score for "thinking that doing extreme things shows the vitality of young people" ($\overline{x}$=2.64). The subjects overwhelmingly wished to have a normal family, job, and life in future ($\overline{x}$=4.39). They had reservations that their parents knew how to teach their children ($\overline{x}$=2.83) and that their schools knew how to teach students ($\overline{x}$=3.28). The subjects cannot be said to have a very low level of self-esteem, as their mean self-esteem score was 31.76, which is at the middle of the scale of 10–50. Their mean depression score was 13.43 on a scale of 0–39, which, according to the simplified version of Beck's Depression Scale, can be interpreted as having a moderate to slightly severe level of depression. Compared with people in their age groups, a majority of subjects considered themselves as being as mature as others ($\overline{x}$=8.38 on a scale of 3–15). Slightly more than half of the subjects had not been stricken by any traumatic or drastic event in the last 30 days. In terms of drug use in the last 30 days, one-third of the subjects did not use drugs, whereas the other two-thirds did.

Looking across the time points, we do not notice many significant changes in the average scores of the variables from T1 to T6. This suggests that psychosocial characteristics, and drug use as well, were quite stable across the six time points.

Selection of Subjects for Analysis

As mentioned above, the sample of subjects were recruited from youth outreach agencies and residential treatment and rehabilitation programmes. For subjects in a residential treatment programme, if they had been in the programme for more than 30 days, they would not have used drugs in the last 30 days in the residential treatment setting, as drug use was prohibited. Thus, not having used drugs in the last 30 days could not reflect the true ability to remain drug-free. Thus, these subjects should not be included in the analysis. On the other hand, if a subject was in a residential programme during the interview but reported drug use in the last 30 days, then he/she might have entered the programme quite recently, and his/her drug use was likely to have occurred before entering the programme. These subjects were included in the analysis. In sum, subjects selected for the present analysis were *those who were either not in a residential T&R programme or were in a residential programme during interview but had reported drug use in the last 30 days.*

Pooled Data and Regression

In order to capitalize on the availability of panel data, which could indicate possible causal influence among the variables, the six waves of data were stacked into an individual time point structure. Not all subjects were able to complete all six interviews. On the average, the subjects received 3.6 interviews across the six time points. The coefficients of the measured predictor variables represented weighted averages of the within-individual (i.e. change over time) and between-individual effects. We used random-effects models, which allow for data that are unbalanced in time by including all respondents in its estimation, regardless of their attrition status or the number of waves they contribute to the individual time point data set (Wooldridge 2002). With the availability of panel data, we were in a much better position to adjust for possibly unobservable variables that affected drug use and other outcomes of interest. For instance, some individuals might be more naturally oriented to abstinence, but others might not be so inclined. Such a feature of the individual could appear as an unmeasured person-specific, time-invariant error component, thus generating heterogeneity bias, which can seriously affect coefficient estimates. The panel nature of the data and the use of random-effects models permit the correction for unmeasured heterogeneity. The possibly unmeasured variables were treated as a random variable and assumed to take a normal distribution, to be time constant, and not to correlate with other measured predictors. An alternative, which was not preferred in this analysis, was to treat the unmeasured variables as fixed effects, which relax the core assumptions by not estimating the effects at all. A caveat of the fixed-effects approach is that time-constant explanatory variables are dropped from the model, and the analysis excludes subjects without outcome variations over time, thereby resulting in a reduction in sample size and loss of efficiency. This is because fixed-effect models are designed to study what causes the dependent variable to change within a given person. A time-invariant characteristic supposedly cannot cause such a change (see Peterson 1993).

Random-effects probit regression analysis (xtprobit in Stata 13.1) was performed to estimate the relative contributions of the independent variables to the binary dependent variable of "drug use in the last 30 days", with the data pooled from T2 to T6 (T1 data did not have any previous time point to compare with and was therefore not included). It should be acknowledged that the binary measurement of drug use is rough. The probit model is a popular specification for a dichotomous response model. It addresses the constraint of the binary measurement by approaching an observed binary outcome as a latent variable: if the latent variable exceeds some value, the observed variable is 1; otherwise it is 0. Applying the probit approach, the drug use outcome was treated as a continuous and latent variable. Although drug use was observed in two states (i.e. drug use versus nondrug use), not all respondents were with the same certainty to take drugs or stay abstinent. One respondent might be very close to the decision of staying drug-free, while another respondent could be very firm in his/her decision. In short, the idea of a latent variable of drug use versus nondrug use is that there is an underlying propensity to be abstinent that produces the observed state of drug use versus being drug free (see Long 1997)

There were a large number of independent variables in the study. Obviously, some of them might not be significantly related to drug use at all six time points. How should independent variables be selected for inclusion in the probit regression? The bivariate association of each independent variable with the dependent variable was examined for each of the six time points. If an independent variable was significantly related to the dependent variable at four or more of the six time points, then this variable would be selected for regression. There was a certain degree of arbitrariness in using "four time points" as the criterion, but "four out of six" already constituted over half of the total number of time points.

References

Agnew, R. (1992). Foundation for a general strain theory of crime and delinquency. *Criminology, 30*, 47–87.

Anderson, T. L. (1993). Types of identity transformation in drug-using and recovery careers. *Sociological Focus, 26*, 133–145.

Beck, A. T., Ward, C. H., Mendelson, M., Mock, J., & Erbaugh, J. (1961). An inventory for measuring depression. *Archives of General Psychiatry, 4*(6), 561–571.

Becker, H. (1963). *Outsiders: Studies in the sociology of deviance*. New York: Free Press.

Benson, J. E. (2014). Reevaluating the subjective weathering hypothesis: Subjective aging, coping resources, and the stress process. *Journal of Health and Social Behavior, 55*, 73–90.

Chan, Y. C. (2012). Acute and chronic toxicity in ketamine abusers in Hong Kong. *Journal of Medical Toxicology, 8*, 267–270.

Chan, K. W. S., Lee, T. K. M., Siu, A. M. H., Wong, D. P. L., Kam, C. M., Tsang, S. K. M., & Chan, C. C. H. (2013). Effects of chronic ketamine use on frontal and medical temporal cognition. *Addictive Behaviors, 38*, 2128–2132.

Cheung, Y. W. (2012). *A longitudinal survey of psychoactive drug abusers in Hong Kong*. Reported submitted to Beat Drugs Fund, Narcotics Division, Security Bureau, Government of the Hong Kong SAR. In website of Narcotics Division: http://www.nd.gov.hk/pdf/Longitudinal%20Survey%20of%20Psychoactive%20Drug%20Abusers%20in%20Hong%20Kong%20-%20report.pdf. Access date: April 9, 2017.

Cheung, Y. W., & Cheung, N. W. T. (2003). Social capital and risk level of posttreatment drug use: Implications for harm reduction among male treated addicts in Hong Kong. *Addiction Research & Theory, 11*(3), 145–162.

Cheung, N. W. T., & Cheung, Y. W. (2006). Is Hong Kong experiencing normalization of adolescent drug use? Some reflections on the normalization thesis. *Substance Use & Misuse, 41*(14), 1967–1990.

Jones, S. P., & Heaven, P. C. L. (1998). Psychosocial correlates of adolescent drug-taking behaviour. *Journal of Adolescence, 21*(2), 127–134.

Liang, H. J., Lau, C. G., Tang, A., Chan, F., Ungvari, G. S., & Tang, W. K. (2013). Cognitive impairments in poly-drug ketamine users. *Addictive Behaviors, 38*(11), 2661–2666.

Liang, H. J., Lau, C. G., Tang, K. L., Chan, F., Ungvari, G. S., & Tang, W. K. (2014). Are sexes affected differently by ketamine? An exploratory study in ketamine users. *Substance Use & Misuse, 49*(4), 395–404.

Long, J. S. (1997). *Regression models for categorical and limited dependent variables*. Thousand Oaks: Sage.

Merton, R. (1957). *Social theory and social structure*. New York: Free Press.

Mok, P. W. K., Wong, W. H. S., Lee, P. W. H., & Low, L. C. K. (2008). Is teenage obesity associated with depression and low self-esteem? A pilot study. *Hong Kong Journal of Paediatrics (New Series), 13*, 30–38.

Moore, S., Laflin, M. T., & Weis, D. L. (1996). The role of cultural norms in the self-esteem and drug use relationship. *Adolescence, 31*, 523–542.

Narcotics Division. (2014). *Central Registry of Drug Abuse sixty-third report (2004–2013)*. Hong Kong: Narcotics Division, Security Bureau, Government of the Hong Kong SAR.

Parker, H., Aldridge, J., & Measham, F. (1998). *Illegal leisure: The normalization of adolescent recreational drug use*. London: Routledge.

Peterson, T. (1993). Recent advances in longitudinal methodology. *Annual Review of Sociology, 19*, 425–512.

Poon, T. L., Wong, K. F., Chan, M. Y., Fung, K. W., Chum, S. K., Man, C. W., et al. (2010). Upper gastrointestinal problems in inhalational ketamine abusers. *Journal of Digestive Diseases, 11*, 106–110.

Rosenberg, M. (1965). *Society and the adolescent self-image*. Princeton: Princeton University Press.

Tam, Y. H., Ng, C. F., Wong, Y. S., Pang, K. K. Y., Hong, Y. L., Lee, W. M., & Lai, P. T. (2016). Population-based survey of the prevalence of lower urinary tract symptoms in adolescents with and without psychotropic substance abuse. *Hong Kong Medical Journal, 22*(Aug. 12 online first), 1–10.

Tang, W. K., Liang, H. J., Lau, C. G., Tang, A., & Ungvari, G. S. (2013). Relationship between cognitive impairment and depressive symptoms in current ketamine users. *Journal of Studies in Alcohol and Drugs, 4*(3), 460–468.

Wang, C., Zheng, D., Xu, J., Lam, W., & Yew, D. T. (2013). Brain damages in ketamine addicts as revealed by magnetic resonance imaging. *Frontiers in Neuroanatomy, 7*, 23.

Wei, Y. B., Yang, J. R., Yin, Z., Guo, Q., Liang, B. L., & Zhou, K. Q. (2013). Genitourinary toxicity of ketamine. *Hong Kong Medical Journal, 19*, 341–348.

Wong, G. L., Tam, Y. H., Ng, C. F., Chan, A. W., Choi, P. C., Chu, W. C., Lai, P. B., Chan, H. L., & Wong, V. W. (2014). Liver injury is common among chronic abusers of ketamine. *Clinical Gastroenterology and Hepatology, 12*, 1759–1762.

Wooldridge, J. (2002). *Economic analysis of cross-section and panel data*. Cambridge, MA: MIT Press.

Yew, D. T. (Ed.). (2015). *Ketamine: Use and abuse*. Boca Raton: CRC Press.

Chapter 3
Socio-demographic and Psychosocial Correlates of Drug Use

The major objective of this study was to find out the socio-demographic and psychosocial variables that affected the continuation or discontinuation of drug use of known psychoactive drug users.[1] The first step was to find the bivariate relationship between each of the two groups of independent variables (socio-demographic and psychosocial variables) and the dependent variable of "drug use in the last 30 days" at each of the six time points. This would allow us to know which independent variables were significantly related to drug use and at how many time points. With such information, we can compare the two groups of variables with respect to their influence on the continuation or discontinuation of drug use. Results of the bivariate relationships would also inform the selection of variables to be included in the regressions according to the above-mentioned criterion of being significantly related to drug use at least at four of the six time points

Bivariate Associations

We first examine the bivariate relationship of each of the socio-demographic, psychosocial, and drug use history variables with drug use in the last 30 days. Results are summarized in Table 3.1.

In order to save space, Table 3.1 reports only those socio-demographic variables that were significantly related to drug use in last 30 days at each time point (based on χ^2 tests). Most of the socio-demographic variables (whether or not a student, marital status, having a religion or not, and housing type) were *not* significant at any of the time points. Gender and age were each significant at only one time point

[1] Two preliminary attempts to analyse the relationships between socio-demographic and psychosocial variables and drug use in the study have previously been made (see Cheung 2015; Cheung et al. 2016).

Y.W. Cheung, N.W.-t. Cheung, *Psychoactive Drug Abuse in Hong Kong*,
Quality of Life in Asia 11, DOI 10.1007/978-981-10-6154-7_3

Table 3.1 T1–T6 bivariate relationships between drug use in last 30 days ('yes" and "no") and socio-demographic variables (only significant ones are reported)

	Used drugs in last 30 days		
Socio-demographic variables	%	n	N
T1			
No significant variables			
T2			
Gender ($p < .05$)			497
M	45.0	136	302
F	54.4	106	195
T3			
No significant variables			
T4			
Age ($p < .05$)			356
14–16	41.7	25	60
17–20	30.8	64	208
21 or over	44.3	39	88
T5			
No significant variables			
T6			
No significant variables			

Significance levels are based on χ^2 tests

(gender at T2, age at T4). Thus, overall speaking, socio-demographic variables were not good predictors of continuation/discontinuation of drug use.

How were the psychosocial variables related to drug use in the last 30 days? Table 3.2 shows the bivariate relationship of each of the psychosocial variables, as well as the drug use history variable, to drug use in the last 30 days (all variables were standardized). Unlike socio-demographic variables, a larger number of psychosocial variables were significantly related to drug use (see Table 3.2).

Psychosocial variables significantly related to drug use at four or more time points were as follows:

- Permissiveness to drug use
- Permissiveness to regular drug use
- Permissiveness to occasional drug use
- Life satisfaction
- Think that doing extreme things shows vitality of young people
- Self-esteem
- Depression
- Stricken by stressful events in the last 6 months

Since the variable of "permissiveness to drug use" was already broken down into regular and occasional drug use, it was not counted here. All these seven variables were significant at all six time points, except stricken by stressful events, which was significant at five time points. The other psychoactive variables and the drug use

Table 3.2 T1–T6 bivariate correlations between drug use in the last 30 days and psychosocial variables and drug use history

	r					
Independent variables	T1	T2	T3	T4	T5	T6
No. of years of drug use	−.280**	−.183**	−.117*	−.025	−.049	.035
Permissiveness to drug use	.374**	.402**	.439**	.294**	.329**	.288**
Permissiveness to regular drug use	.313**	293**	.327**	.235**	.274**	179**
Permissiveness to occasional drug use	.406**	.419**	.437**	.323**	.332**	.287**
Level of disappointment if aspired education level not achieved	−.022	−.013	.053	.044	.024	.019
Ever been discriminated by other people	−.126**	−.118**	−.012	.030	.023	.157**
Sense of uncertainty about future	.023	.126**	.081	.200**	.084	.140*
Think that doing extreme things shows the vitality of young people	.118**	.125**	.121**	.239**	.243**	.129*
Wish to have own family, job, and normal life in future	−.072*	−.051	−.044	.012	−.103	−.074
Think that parents don't know how to teach children	−.026	−.027	−.098*	.091	.095	.099
Think that school doesn't know how to teach students	.148**	.057	.057	.030	.158**	.056
Life satisfaction	.254**	−.287**	−.301**	−.377**	−.387**	−.269**
Self-esteem	−.089*	−.115**	−.173**	−.292**	−.271**	−.242**
Depression	.142**	.158**	.201**	.372**	.346**	.359**
Stricken by stressful events	.077*	.058	.102*	.171**	.210**	.164**
Subjective weathering	.077*	.038	.067	.011	.115*	.040

*$p < .05$; **$p < .01$
All variables are standardized

history variable were significantly related to drug use at only three or less time points.

Overall, compared with socio-demographic variables, psychosocial variables were much more significantly related to drug use in the last 30 days. The finding of lack of relationship between socio-demographic characteristics and drug use is not unsettling. The "normalization of recreational drug use" thesis discussed above maintains that the increasing involvement of young people in recreational drug use today is reflected by not only the rise of prevalence of, and growing permissive attitude towards, drug use but also by drug use cutting across gender, age, occupation, socioeconomic condition, and other socio-demographic divisions (Parker et al.1998; Cheung and Cheung 2006). If the initiation of drug use is not affected by socio-demographic characteristics, it is not surprising that the continuation or discontinuation of drug use is not socio-demographically determined.

After comparing the bivariate relationships between the two groups of independent variables and drug use in the last 30 days, our next attempt is to perform probit regression analysis to explain drug use, using only psychosocial variables, due to the absence of socio-demographic variables that were significantly related to drug use at four or more time points.

Explaining Continuation/Discontinuation of Drug Use with Psychosocial Variables

The above-mentioned seven psychosocial variables (permissiveness to regular drug use, permissiveness to occasional drug use, life satisfaction, thinking that doing extreme thing shows vitality of young people, self-esteem, depression, and stricken by stressful events in the last 6 months) were each significantly related to drug use in the last 30 days for five or six time points, and so they satisfied the criterion of selection (significant at four or more time points) and were included in the regression analysis. We first examine the regression results for drug use in the last 30 days as the outcome variable.

Drug Use in Last 30 Days as Outcome Variable

Table 3.3 shows the results of the random-effects probit regression with drug use in the last 30 days as the dependent variable.

There were three types of independent variables in Table 3.3. The first type was the time points of T3–T6, showing whether or not there was any effect due to time. The second type of independent variables was the selected psychosocial variables at the same, or concurrent, time point. The third type was the same set of psychosocial variables at the previous time point (represented by "−1"), which could show the causal effects of the independent variables, if any. Model 1 contained only time points and psychosocial variables at the concurrent time point as independent variables, whereas Model 2 contained not only time points and psychosocial variables at the concurrent time point but also psychosocial variables at the previous time

Table 3.3 Random-effects probit models of drug use in the last 30 days ("yes" or "no") on selected psychosocial variables based on data pooled from T2 to T6

	Model 1 ($N = 1997$)		Model 2 ($N = 1881$)	
Independent variables	β	S.E.	β	S.E.
T3	−.176	.113	−.037	.106
T4	−.077	.120	.092	.117
T5	−.368	.129	−.111	.126
T6	−.271	.142	−.005	.136
Concurrent time point				
Permissiveness to regular drug use	.357**	.055	.270**	.050
Permissiveness to occasional drug use	.644***	.068	.438***	.064
Think that doing extreme things shows the vitality of young people	.009	.052	−.011	.047
Life satisfaction	−.436***	.057	−.350***	.051
Self-esteem	−.005	.067	−.049	.062
Depression	.216**	.063	.140 *	.058
Stricken by stressful events	.065	.046	.061	.041
Previous time point				
Drug use in the last 30 days (−1)			471***	.054
Permissiveness to regular drug use (−1)			.003	.049
Permissiveness to occasional drug use (−1)			−.052	.060
Think that doing extreme things shows the vitality of young people (−1)			.025	.046
Life satisfaction (−1)			−.012	.050
Self-esteem (−1)			−.135*	.060
Depression (−1)			.034	.058
Stricken by stressful events (−1)			.046	.042
Log likelihood	−910.99		−823.34	
Wald chi-square	257.31***		411.80***	
df	11		19	
Rho	.562***		244***	

* $p < .05$; ** $p < .01$; *** $p < .001$
All βs are standardized probit coefficients
Rho is the proportion of the total variance explained by the panel-level variance. A significant Rho means that there is enough variability between individuals to favour a random-effects probit regression (a panel estimator) over a standard probit regression (a pooled estimator)

point (−1). Here, "drug use in the last 30 days (−1)" was also added in order to ascertain its causal effect on drug use in last 30 day at the current time point.

In Table 3.3, all the time points did not yield any significant regression coefficients, suggesting that the relationships between the psychosocial variables and drug use in last 30 days did not significantly vary across different time points. At the concurrent time point (Model 1), permissiveness to regular drug use, permissiveness to occasional drug use, life satisfaction, and depression were significantly related to drug use in the last 30 days. When psychosocial variables and drug use in the last 30 days at the previous time point were added to the regression (Model 2), the same psychosocial variables at the concurrent time point were significant, and the effects of variables from the previous time point came from drug use in the last 30 days (−1) and self-esteem (−1). In Model 2, at the same time point, the strongest influence on drug use in last 30 days came from permissiveness to occasional drug use ($\beta = .438$, $p < .001$). The influence of permissiveness to regular drug use was smaller but still quite strong ($\beta = .270$, $p < .01$). Another strong variable was life satisfaction ($\beta = -.350$, $p < .001$). Depression was also significantly related, although not as strong as the other three variables ($\beta = .140$, $p < .05$). As to effects of the two significant variables from the previous time point, drug use in the last 30 days (−1) yielded a β coefficient of .471 ($p < .001$), and self-esteem (−1) produced a β of −.135 ($p < .05$).

In sum, the dependent variable of drug use in the last 30 days was significantly affected by the two permissive attitudes towards drug use (regular and occasional use), life satisfaction, and depression at the same time point. The more permissive the attitude towards regular or occasional drug use, the lower the life satisfaction, and the higher the depression level, the more likely that drug use had occurred in the last 30 days. Variables in the previous time point that also affected drug use were drug use (−1) and self-esteem (−1). Subjects who had used a drug at the previous time point, and those having a lower level of self-esteem at the previous time point, were more likely to have used a drug in the last 30 days at the current time point.

After conducting a regression analysis of the dependent variable of drug use in the last 30 days to find out which psychosocial variables significantly affected it, we would like to next explore how the psychosocial variables significantly related to drug use were affected by other psychosocial variables as well as socio-demographic ones. Before we conducted a regression analysis for each of the significant psychosocial variables, we followed the procedures of selection of independent variables—checking the bivariate relationships of each of the socio-demographic and psychosocial variables with drug use and selecting those that were significant at four or more time points. For socio-demographic variables, it has been shown earlier that none of them met the criterion of being significantly related to drug use at four or more time points. Thus, we only included gender, age, and student status in the bivariate checks. In addition, drug use history (number of years of drug use) was also included.

Since a permissive attitude towards drug use has been found to be a powerful predictor of continuous drug use in Hong Kong,[2] and since attitude-behaviour is a well-recognized link in social science research, we treat the two permissive attitudes as intervening variables between the other psychosocial or demographic variables and drug use in the last 30 days. We next conducted a regression analysis of how the other psychosocial variables might affect the two permissiveness variables, followed by life satisfaction, self-esteem, and depression. It should be noted here that

[2] For example, a study of 504 marginal youths and 503 regular secondary school students in Hong Kong in 2002–2004 found that the level of permissiveness to drug use of the marginal youths (80% of them had previously taken drugs) was six times higher than that of regular students (Cheung and Cheung 2006).

in the bivariate check and regression analysis of each of the two permissiveness variables, the other permissiveness variable would not be included, due to the very high correlation between the two variables.

Permissiveness to Regular Drug Use as Outcome Variable

Bivariate correlations of other psychosocial variables, the three socio-demographic variables (gender, age, student status), and number of years of drug use with drug use in the last 30 days were presented in Table 3.4.

Independent variables that had yielded significant bivariate relationships with permissiveness to regular drug use at four or more time points were gender, think that doing extreme things shows vitality of young people, wish to have normal life in future, life satisfaction, self-esteem, and depression. These variables were included in the random-effects ordered probit regression analysis. Table 3.5 shows the results of the regression.

At the concurrent time point (Model 1), independent variables that were significantly related to permissiveness to regular drug use were think that doing extreme things shows vitality of young people, wish to have normal life in future, life satisfaction, and self-esteem. Depression did not yield a significant regression coefficient. In Model 2, which included both concurrent and previous time points, the same set of variables at the concurrent time point in Model 1 were significant. Think that doing extreme things shows vitality of young people yielded the strongest coefficient ($\beta = .270$, $p < .001$), followed by sex ($\beta = .231$, $p < .01$), wish to have normal life in future ($\beta = -.187$, $p < .001$), and self-esteem ($\beta = -.185$, $p < .001$). Life satisfaction was also significantly related, although its coefficient was smaller than those of the other variables ($\beta = -.085$, $p < .05$).

The socio-demographic variable of gender yielded a significant regression coefficient in both Model 1 ($\beta = .297$, $p < .01$) and Model 2 ($\beta = .231$, $p < .01$). As to effects from variables in the previous time point, variables that had significant effects were drug use in last 30 days (−1) ($\beta = .138$, $p < .001$), permissiveness to regular drug use (−1) ($\beta = .160$, $p < .001$), and self-esteem (−1) ($\beta = -.142$, $p < .01$). However, life satisfaction (−1) and depression (−1) did not have significant effects on permissiveness to regular drug use at the concurrent time point.

The 6th time point yielded a significant regression coefficient in Model 1 ($\beta = -.238$, $p < .05$). This was an indication that the change in sample characteristics at T6 was significantly related to drug use in the last 30 days at T6. This result was not unsettling. One of the reasons for the occurrence of changes in the characteristics of the sample was that more and more subjects left the study at later time points and there was a higher tendency for drug-using subjects to drop out. Regardless of changes in the sample characteristics, the relationships among the variables were not affected. When effects of variables at the previous time points were also considered (Model 2), T6 was no longer significant.

Table 3.4 T1–T6 bivariate correlations between permissiveness to regular drug use and socio-demographic, drug use history, and psychosocial variables

	r					
Independent variables	T1	T2	T3	T4	T5	T6
Gender (1 = male; 2 = female)	.149**	.135**	.108*	.045	.133*	.073
Age	−.147**	−.071	−.005	−.054	−.051	.069
Student versus non-student status	.012	−.030	−.106*	−.039	.011	.011
No. of years of drug use	−.138**	−.060	−.052	−.124*	−.075	.036
Level of disappointment if aspired education level is not achieved	−.102**	−.140**	.020	−.130*	−.097	−.060
Ever been discriminated by other people	−.098**	−.104**	−.062	−.055	−.090	−.032
Sense of uncertainty about future	.016	.151**	.029	.057	.015	−.040
Think that doing extreme things shows vitality of young people	252**	.317**	.352**	.350**	.366**	.165**
Wish to have own family, job, and normal life in future	−.144**	−.130**	−.198**	−.175**	−.283**	−.287**
Think that parents don't know how to teach children	.023	.045	.006	.150**	−.008	.147*
Think that school doesn't know how to teach students	.127**	.070	.057	.096	.172**	.061
Life satisfaction	−.140**	−.212**	−.109*	−.124*	−.184**	−.041
Self-esteem	−.040	−.125**	−.100**	−.161**	−.159**	−.161**
Depression	.095**	.096*	.066	.107*	.108*	.121*
Stricken by stressful events	.020	−.051	.071	.024	.090	−.014
Subjective weathering (compare maturity)	.042	.031	.039	.007	.086	.005

$^{*}p < .05$; $^{**}p < .01$

Table 3.5 Random-effects ordered probit models of permissiveness to regular drug use on selected socio-demographic and psychosocial variables based on data pooled from T2 to T6

	Model 1 ($N = 2009$)		Model 2 ($N = 1896$)	
Independent variables	β	S.E.	β	S.E.
T3	−.026	.080	.010	.081
T4	−.056	.084	−.007	.089
T5	−.109	.087	−.056	.093
T6	−.238*	.096	−.138	.100
Gender (1 = male; 2 = female)	.297**	.089	.231**	.081
Concurrent time point				
Think that doing extreme things shows vitality of young people	.328***	.035	.270***	.036
Wish to have own family, job, and normal life in future	−.200***	.032	−.187***	.032
Life satisfaction	−.110**	.039	−.085*	.039
Self-esteem	−.117*	.046	−.185***	.049
Depression	−.061	.044	−.041	.045
Previous time point				
Drug use in the last 30 days (−1)			.138 ***	.036
Permissiveness to regular drug use (−1)			.160 ***	.041
Think that doing extreme things shows the vitality of young people (−1)			.064	.035
Wish to have own family, job, and normal life in future (−1)			−.055	.033
Life satisfaction (−1)			−.004	.039
Self-esteem (−1)			−.142**	.047
Depression (−1)			−.026	.045
Log likelihood	−1729.00		−1597.84	
Wald chi-square	194.74***		268.30***	
df	10		17	
Panel-level variance	.547***		331***	

*$p < .05$; **$p < .01$; ***$p < .001$
All βs are standardized ordered probit coefficients
The significance of the panel-level variance means that there is sufficient variability between individuals to favour a random-effects ordered probit regression (a panel estimator) over a standard ordered probit regression (a pooled estimator)

Permissiveness to Occasional Drug Use as Outcome Variable

Table 3.6 shows the bivariate relationships between independent variables and permissiveness to occasional drug use at the six time points.

Seven of the independent variables were significantly related to permissiveness to occasional drug use at four or more time points: gender, number of years of drug use, think that doing extreme things shows vitality of young people, think that

Table 3.6 T1–T6 bivariate correlations between permissiveness to occasional drug use and socio-demographic, drug use history, and psychosocial variables

	r					
Independent variables	T1	T2	T3	T4	T5	T6
Gender (1 = male; 2 = female)	.186**	.155**	.196**	.173**	.158**	.101
Age	−.233**	−.102*	−.125**	−.062	−.051	.065
Non-student versus student status	.021	.008	−.029	−.005	−.016	−.045
No. of years of drug use	−.265**	−.183**	−.173**	−.163**	−.137*	−.020
Level of disappointment if aspired education level is not achieved	−.138**	−.144**	−.037	−.059	−.055	−.045
Ever been discriminated by other people	−.135**	−.036	−.037	−.101*	−.024	−.003
Sense of uncertainty about future	.045	.183**	219**	.136**	.069	.085
Think that doing extreme things shows the vitality of young people	.340**	.368**	.394**	.379**	.387**	.204**
Wish to have own family, job, and normal life in future	−.129**	−.071	−.090	−.079	−.217**	−.216**
Think that parents don't know how to teach children	.039	.042	.094	.075	.062	.077
Think that school doesn't know how to teach students	.208**	.216**	.125**	.018	.176**	.075
Life satisfaction	−.141**	−.240**	−260**	−.226**	−.212**	−.051
Self-esteem	.020	−.103**	−.135**	−.156**	−.196**	−.222**
Depression	.095**	.148**	.196**	.151**	.155**	.174**
Stricken by stressful events	.020	.059	.158**	.043	.103	.055
Subjective weathering	.100*	0.039	0.099*	0.042	0.109*	−0.024

*$p < .05$; **$p < .01$

school doesn't know how to teach students, life satisfaction, self-esteem, and depression.

Ordered probit regression results are shown in Table 3.7. In Model 1, where only concurrent time point is considered, gender, number of years of drug use, think that doing extreme things shows vitality of young people, think that school doesn't know how to teach students, and life satisfaction were significantly related to

Table 3.7 Random-effects ordered probit models of permissiveness to occasional drug use on selected socio-demographic, drug use history, and psychosocial variables based on data pooled from T2 to T6

	Model 1 (N = 1867)		Model 2 (N = 1687)	
Independent variables	β	S.E.	β	S.E.
T3	−.121	.074	.017	.073
T4	−.331***	.089	−.118	.089
T5	−.457***	.083	−.173	.095
T6	−.603***	.092	−.212*	.091
Gender (1 = male; 2 = female)	.363**	.110	.192*	.070
No. of years of drug use	−.182***	.046	−.010	.033
Concurrent time point				
Think that doing extreme things shows the vitality of young people	.383***	.036	310***	.034
Think that school doesn't know how to teach students	.087**	.034	.087**	.031
Life satisfaction	−.128 **	.039	−.109**	.036
Self-esteem	−.067	.047	−.097*	.044
Depression	.061	.045	.024	.042
Previous time point				
Drug use in the last 30 days (−1)			141***	.034
Permissiveness to occasional drug use (−1)			584***	.047
Think that doing extreme things shows the vitality of young people (−1)			−.017	.035
Think that school doesn't know how to teach students (−1)			.026	.031
Life satisfaction (−1)			−.037	.036
Self-esteem (−1)			−.150***	.042
Depression (−1)			−.045	.041
Log likelihood	−2608.21		−2259.26	
Wald chi-square	287.89***		646.54***	
df	11		18	
Panel-level variance	1.112***		.155**	

* $p < .05$; ** $p < .01$; *** $p < .001$
All β s are standardized ordered probit coefficients
The significance of the panel-level variance means that there is sufficient variability between individuals to favour a random-effects ordered pro bit regression (a panel estimator) over a standard ordered probit regression (a pooled estimator)

permissiveness to occasional drug use. In Model 2, these variables, except number of years of drug use, also yielded significant coefficients at the concurrent time point. Think that doing extreme things shows vitality of young people was most strongly related to permissiveness to occasional drug use (β = .310, $p < .001$), followed by gender (β = .192, $p < .05$), life satisfaction (β = −.109, $p < .01$), self-esteem (β = −.097, $p < .05$), and think that school does not know how to teach students (β = .087, $p < .01$). Variables in the previous time point that had significant effects on permissiveness to occasional drug use were drug use in the last 30 days (−1) ($\beta = .141$, $p < .001$), permissiveness to occasional drug use (−1) ($\beta = .584$, $p < .001$), and self-esteem (−1) ($\beta = -.150$, $p < .001$).

Like in the regression of permissiveness to regular drug use, there were time points that were significant (T4, T5, and T6). Changes in sampling characteristics over time (due to drop-out cases, etc.) at these time points had affected permissiveness to occasional drug use, but they did not affect the relationships among the variables.

Life Satisfaction as Outcome Variable

Table 3.8 shows the variables that had significant bivariate relationships with life satisfaction at four or more time points.

These variables included permissiveness to regular drug use, permissiveness to occasional drug use, ever been discriminated by other people, sense of uncertainty about future, think that doing extreme things shows vitality of young people, think that parents don't know how to teacher children, think that schools don't know how to teach students, self-esteem, depression, and stricken by stressful events.

The regression results are shown in Table 3.9. At the concurrent time point (Model 1), permissiveness to occasional drug use, ever been discriminated by other people, uncertainty about future, self-esteem, depression, and stricken by stressful events were significant. In Model 2, permissiveness to occasional drug use ($\beta = -.107$, $p < .05$), ever been discriminated by other people ($\beta = -.073$, $p < .05$), sense of uncertainty about future ($\beta = -.106$, $p < .01$), self-esteem ($\beta = .350$, $p < .001$), and depression ($\beta = -.317$, $p < .001$) were significant at the concurrent time point. Life satisfaction (−1) ($\beta = .369$, $p < .001$), depression (−1) ($\beta = .090$, $p < .05$), and stricken by stressful events (−1) ($\beta = .073$, $p < .05$) were variables at the previous time point that had significant effects on life satisfaction.

Self-Esteem as Outcome Variable

There was a long list of independent variables that self-esteem has significant bivariate relationships with (Table 3.10):

- Gender
- Permissiveness to regular drug use
- Permissiveness to occasional drug use
- Disappointment if aspired education level not achieved
- Ever been discriminated by other people
- Sense of uncertainty about future
- Think that doing extreme things shows vitality of young people

Table 3.8 T1–T6 bivariate correlations between life satisfaction and socio-demographic, drug use history, and psychosocial variables

	r					
Independent variables	T1	T2	T3	T4	T5	T6
Gender (1 = male; 2 = female)	–.083*	–.007	–.031	–.041	–.103	–.144*
Age	.073*	–.036	–.006	–.029	.011	–.045
Student versus non-student status	.031	.051	.065	.035	.037	.017
No. of years of drug use	.155**	.045	.070	.003	.074	.005
Permissiveness to occasional drug use	–.141*	–.240*	–.260*	–.226*	–.212*	–.051
Permissiveness to regular drug use	–.140*	–.212*	–.109*	–.124*	–.184*	–.042
Level of disappointment if aspired education level is not achieved	–.080*	–.038	–.080	–.080	–.162**	–.121*
Ever been discriminated by other people	–.086*	–.131**	–.166**	–.096	–.053	–.225**
Sense of uncertainty about future	–.209**	–.265**	–.298**	–.315**	–.221**	–.270**
Think that doing extreme things shows the vitality of young people	.014	–.133**	–.146**	–.120**	–.089	–.135**
Wish to have own family, job, and normal life in future	.025	.037	.060	.086	.084	.090
Think that parents don't know how to teach children	–.172**	–.183**	–.169**	–.224**	–.194**	–.140*
Think that school doesn't know how to teach students	–.158**	–.199**	–.111**	–.018	–.189**	–.127*
Self-esteem	.340**	.451**	.431**	.508**	.442**	.560**
Depression	–.367**	–.476**	–.420**	–.515**	–.502**	–.542**
Stricken by stressful events	–.122**	–.169**	–.106**	–.146**	–.224**	–.171**
Subjective weathering	–.024	.042	–.012	.096	.071	.175*

*$p < .05$; **$p < .01$

Table 3.9 Random-effects ordered probit models of life satisfaction on selected psychosocial variables based on data pooled from T2 to T6

	Model 1 (N = 1869)		Model 2 (N = 1679)	
	β	S.E.	β	S.E.
T3	−0.035	(0.075)	−0.044	(0.075)
T4	−0.091	(0.090)	−0.127	(0.091)
T5	−0.031	(0.082)	−0.101	(0.096)
T6	−0.065	(0.091)	−0.090	(0.090)
Concurrent time point				
Permissiveness to regular drug use	−0.055	(0.038)	−0.048	(0.036)
Permissiveness to occasional drug use	−0.147***	(0.042)	−0.107*	(0.043)
Ever been discriminated by other people	−0.052	(0.036)	−0.073*	(0.035)
Sense of uncertainty about future	−0.089**	(0.034)	−0.106**	(0.033)
Think that doing extreme things shows the vitality of young people	−0.014	(0.035)	−0.011	(0.035)
Think that parents don't know how to teach children	−0.065	(0.035)	−0.024	(0.036)
Think that school doesn't know how to teach students	−0.044	(0.033)	−0.050	(0.032)
Self-esteem	0.425***	(0.044)	0.350***	(0.046)
Depression	−0.349***	(0.044)	−0.317***	(0.044)
Stricken by stressful events	−0.088**	(0.033)	−0.048	(0.032)
Previous time point				
Drug use in the last 30 days (−1)			−0.014	(0.034)
Life satisfaction (−1)			0.369***	(0.046)
Permissiveness to regular drug use (−1)			0.027	(0.035)
Permissiveness to occasional drug use (−1)			−0.020	(0.042)
Ever been discriminated by other people (−1)			0.023	(0.034)
Sense of uncertainty about future (−1)			−0.035	(0.033)
Think that doing extreme things shows the vitality of young people (−1)			−0.013	(0.034)
Think that parents don't know how to teach children (−1)			−0.035	(0.036)
Think that school doesn't know how to teach students (−1)			0.015	(0.032)
Self-esteem (−1)			−0.060	(0.043)
Depression (−1)			0.090*	(0.043)
Stricken by stressful events (−1)			0.073*	(0.030)
Log likelihood	−2160.91		−1811.98	
Wald chi-square	466.42***		615.09***	
df	14		26	
Panel-level variance	.445***		.085*	

*$p < .05$; **$p < .01$; ***$p < .001$

All β s are standardized ordered probit coefficients

The significance of the panel-level variance means that there is sufficient variability between individuals to favour a random-effects ordered pro bit regression (a panel estimator) over a standard ordered probit regression (a pooled estimator)

Table 3.10 T1–T6 bivariate correlations between self-esteem and socio-demographic, drug use history, and psychosocial variables

	r					
Independent variables	T1	T2	T3	T4	T5	T6
Gender (1 = male; 2 = female)	−.124*	−.122*	−.091	−.141*	−.132*	−.206*
Age	−.055	−.003	.018	−.023	.029	−.028
Student versus non-student status	.008	.057	.043	.074	.120*	−.018
No. of years of drug use	−.089*	−.062	−.068	.037	.084	−.004
Permissiveness to occasional drug use	.020	−.103*	−.135*	−.156*	−.196*	−.222*
Permissiveness to regular drug use	−.040	−.125*	−.101*	−.161*	−.159*	−.161*
Level of disappointment if aspired education level is not achieved	−.170*	−.094*	−.153*	−.198*	−.212*	−.183*
Ever been discriminated by other people	−.193*	−.125*	−.123*	−.134*	−.077	−.260*
Sense of uncertainty about future	−.291*	−.270*	−.401*	−.420*	−.337*	−.342*
Think that doing extreme things shows vitality of young people	−.005	−.083*	−.131*	−.160*	−.245*	−.198*
Wish to have normal life in future	.065	.048	.108*	.136*	.165*	.193*
Think that parents don't know how to teach children	−.115*	−.188*	−.129*	−.158*	−.167*	−.216*
Think that school doesn't know how to teach students	.042	−.105*	−.049	−.034	−.097	−.138*
Life satisfaction	.340*	.451*	.431*	.508*	.442*	.560*
Depression	−.577*	−.577*	−.590*	−.640*	−.614*	−.655*
Stricken by drastic events	−.125*	−.113*	−.104*	−.095	−.111*	−.164*
Subjective weathering	.221*	.202*	.172*	.194*	.185*	.199*

*$p < .05$

- Wish to have normal life in future
- Think that parents don't know how to teach children
- Life satisfaction
- Depression
- Stricken by stressful events
- Subjective weathering

These variables were included in the regression analysis, and the results of which are shown in Table 3.11.

A large number of psychosocial variables significantly affected self-esteem (Table 3.11). When only concurrent time point was considered (Model 1), variables that were significantly related to self-esteem were permissiveness to regular drug

Table 3.11 Random-effects maximum likelihood linear models of self-esteem on selected psychosocial variables based on data pooled from T2 to T6

	Model 1 (N = 1796)		Model 2 (N = 1571)	
	β	S.E.	β	S.E.
T3	0.030	(0.037)	0.029	(0.043)
T4	0.073	(0.039)	0.025	(0.047)
T5	0.042	(0.041)	-0.029	(0.049)
T6	0.097*	(0.045)	0.045	(0.052)
Gender (1 = male; 2 = female)	−0.043	(0.052)	0.016	(0.037)
Concurrent time point				
Permissiveness to regular drug use	−0.069***	(0.019)	−0.059**	(0.020)
Permissiveness to occasional drug use	0.014	(0.022)	−0.014	(0.023)
Level of disappointment if aspired education level is not achieved	−0.073***	(0.017)	−0.046**	(0.018)
Ever been discriminated by other people	−0.011	(0.018)	0.008	(0.019)
Sense of uncertainty about future	−0.117***	(0.017)	−0.116***	(0.018)
Think that doing extreme things shows vitality of young people	−0.017	(0.018)	−0.035	(0.019)
Wish to have own family, job, and normal life in future	0.060***	(0.015)	0.079***	(0.016)
Think that parents don't know how to teach children	−0.021	(0.018)	−0.018	(0.019)
Life satisfaction	0.166***	(0.018)	0.142***	(0.020)
Depression	−0.394***	(0.021)	−0.374***	(0.022)
Stricken by stressful events	0.017	(0.016)	0.024	(0.018)
Subjective weathering	−0.058**	(0.018)	−0.034	(0.019)
Previous time point				
Drug use in the last 30 days (−1)			0.027	(0.019)
Self-esteem (−1)			0.405***	(0.038)
Permissiveness to regular drug use (−1)			0.028	(0.020)
Permissiveness to occasional drug use (−1)			0.012	(0.023)
Level of disappointment if aspired education level is not achieved (−1)			−0.001	(0.018)
Ever been discriminated by other people (−1)			−0.009	(0.018)
Sense of uncertainty about future (−1)			0.035	(0.019)
Think that doing extreme things shows vitality of young people (−1)			0.021	(0.019)
Wish to have own family, job, and normal life in future (−1)			−0.028	(0.017)
Think that parents don't know how to teach children (−1)			0.017	(0.019)
Life satisfaction (−1)			−0.022	(0.020)

(continued)

Table 3.11 (continued)

	Model 1 ($N = 1796$)		Model 2 ($N = 1571$)	
	β	S.E.	β	S.E.
Depression (−1)			0.051*	(0.026)
Stricken by stressful events (−1)			0.042*	(0.017)
Subjective weathering (−1)			−0.006	(0.019)
Log likelihood	−1732.70		−1447.37	
Likelihood ratio chi-square	883.43***		928.18	
df	17		31	
Rho	.476***		.086*	

Standard errors in parentheses
* $p < .05$; ** $p < .01$; *** $p < .001$
All βs are standardized coefficients
Rho is the proportion of the total variance explained by the panel-level variance. A significant Rho means that there is enough variability between individuals to favour a random-effects probit regression (a panel estimator) over a standard probit regression (a pooled estimator)

use, disappointed if aspired education level is not achieved, sense of uncertainty about future, wishing to have own family, job, and normal life in future, life satisfaction, depression, and subjective weathering. When the previous time point was also considered (Model 2), all of these psychosocial variables at the concurrent time point, except subjective weathering, were still significant. Beta coefficients yielded by these psychosocial variables were −.059 ($p < .01$) for permissiveness to regular drug use, −.046 ($p < .01$) for disappointed if aspired education level is not achieved, −.116 ($p < .001$) for sense of uncertainty about future, .079 ($p < .001$) for wishing to have own family, job, and normal life in future, .142 ($p < .001$) for life satisfaction, and −.374 ($p < .001$) for depression.

Psychosocial variables in the previous time point that had significant effects of self-esteem were self-esteem itself (−1), with a very strong beta coefficient of .405 ($p < .001$). Depression (−1) and stricken by stressful events (−1) at previous time point were also significant, although the beta coefficients were small (.051, $p < .05$ for depression −1; .042, $p < .05$ for stricken by stressful events −1).

Depression as Outcome Variable

Depression was also correlated with a large number of independent variables at four or more time points (Table 3.12):

- Gender
- Permissiveness of regular drug use
- Permissiveness to occasional drug use
- Disappointment if aspired education level not achieved
- Ever been discriminated by other people
- Sense of uncertainty about future
- Think that doing extreme things shows vitality of young people

Table 3.12 T1–T6 bivariate correlations between depression and socio-demographic, drug use history, and psychosocial variables

	r					
Independent variables	T1	T2	T3	T4	T5	T6
Gender (1 = male; 2 = female)	.157*	.137*	.089	.122*	.135*	.230*
Age	−.027	.053	−.065	.035	.036	.002
Student versus non-student status	.004	−.062	.037	−.006	−.029	.004
No. of years of drug use	.024	.064	.036	.058	−.016	.016
Permissiveness to occasional drug use	.099*	.148*	.196*	.151*	.155*	.174*
Permissiveness to regular drug use	.095*	.096*	.066	.107*	.108*	.121*
Level of disappointment if aspired education level is not achieved	.199*	.061	.209*	.157*	.158*	.182*
Ever been discriminated by other people	.265*	.229*	.255*	.281*	.184*	.274*
Sense of uncertainty about future	.279*	.321*	.447*	.426*	.363*	.373*
Think that doing extreme things shows vitality of young people	.107*	.143*	.162*	.171*	.125*	.156*
Wish to have normal life in future	.006	.006	.067	−.020	−.047	.026
Think that parents don't know how to teach children	.212*	.251*	.262*	.251*	.256*	.215*
Think that school doesn't know how to teach students	.132*	.190*	.176*	.053	.252*	.254*
Life satisfaction	−.367*	−.476*	−.420*	−.515*	−.502*	−.542*
Self-esteem	−.577*	−.577*	−.590*	−.640*	−.614*	−.655*
Stricken by drastic events	.246*	.227*	.272*	.263*	.283*	.318*
Subjective weathering	−.141*	−.121*	−.014	−.038	−.108*	−.116*

*$p < .05$

- Think that parents don't know how to teach children
- Think that school doesn't know how to teach students
- Life satisfaction
- Self-esteem
- Stricken by stressful events
- Subjective weathering

Results of the regression containing these independent variables are shown in Table 3.13.

In Table 3.13, significant variables at the concurrent time point (Model 1) that affected depression were gender, ever been discriminated by other people, sense of uncertainty about future, think that parents don't know how to teach children, think

Table 3.13 Random-effects maximum likelihood linear models of depression on selected psychosocial variables based on data pooled from T2 to T6

	Model 1 ($N = 1691$)		Model 2 ($N = 1413$)	
	β	S.E	β	S.E.
T3	−0.102**	(0.040)	−0.054	(0.045)
T4	−0.051	(0.048)	0.014	(0.055)
T5	−0.094*	(0.044)	−0.012	(0.057)
T6	−0.035	(0.048)	0.071	(0.055)
Gender (1 = male; 2 = female)	0.128**	(0.046)	0.072	(0.038)
Concurrent time point				
Permissiveness to regular drug use	−0.021	(0.020)	−0.015	(0.021)
Permissiveness to occasional drug use	0.037	(0.022)	0.022	(0.025)
Level of disappointment if aspired education level is not achieved	0.018	(0.018)	0.035	(0.019)
Ever been discriminated by other people	0.073***	(0.019)	0.071***	(0.021)
Sense of uncertainty about future	0.093***	(0.018)	0.096***	(0.019)
Think that doing extreme things shows vitality of young people	0.034	(0.019)	0.031	(0.021)
Think that parents don't know how to teach children	0.055**	(0.019)	0.048*	(0.021)
Think that school doesn't know how to teach students	0.058***	(0.017)	0.036	(0.019)
Life satisfaction	−0.157***	(0.020)	−0.152***	(0.021)
Self-esteem	−0.421***	(0.022)	−0.389***	(0.025)
Stricken by stressful events	0.118***	(0.017)	0.113***	(0.019)
Subjective weathering	0.006	(0.018)	0.017	(0.020)
Previous time point				
Drug use in the last 30 days (−1)			0.020	(0.020)
Depression (−1)			0.307***	(0.034)
Permissiveness to regular drug use (−1)			0.028	(0.021)
Permissiveness to occasional drug use (−1)			−0.003	(0.025)
Level of disappointment if aspired education level is not achieved (−1)			0.001	(0.019)
Ever been discriminated by other people (−1)			−0.019	(0.020)
Sense of uncertainty about future (−1)			−0.019	(0.020)
Think that doing extreme things shows vitality of young people (−1)			−0.005	(0.020)
Think that parents don't know how to teach children (−1)			−0.001	(0.021)
Think that school doesn't know how to teach students (−1)			0.025	(0.019)
Life satisfaction (−1)			0.035	(0.022)

(continued)

Table 3.13 (continued)

	Model 1 ($N = 1691$)		Model 2 ($N = 1413$)	
	β	S.E	β	S.E.
Self-esteem (−1)			0.113***	(0.026)
Stricken by stressful events (−1)			0.035	(0.018)
Subjective weathering (−1)			−0.016	(0.020)
Log likelihood	−1673.41		−1345.57	
Likelihood ratio chi-square	887.68***		871.69	
df	17		31	
Rho	.310***		.05	

* $p < .05$; ** $p < .01$; *** $p < .001$
All βs are standardized probit coefficients
Rho is the proportion of the total variance explained by the panel-level variance. A significant Rho means that there is enough variability between individuals to favour a random-effects probit regression (a panel estimator) over a standard probit regression (a pooled estimator)

that school doesn't know how to teach students, life satisfaction, self-esteem, and stricken by stressful events. In Model 2, when previous time point was also considered in the regression, gender and think that school doesn't know how to teach students at the concurrent time point became non-significant. Those that remained significant at the concurrent time point were ever been discriminated by other people (β = .071, $p < .001$), sense of uncertainty about future (β = .096, $p < .001$), think that parents don't know how to teach children (β = .048, $p < .05$), life satisfaction (β = −.152, $p < .001$), self-esteem (β = −.389, $p < .001$), and stricken by stressful events (β = .113, $p < .001$). Significant independent variables at the previous time point that affected depression included depression itself (−1) (β = .307, $p < .001$) and self-esteem (−1) (β = .113, $p < .001$).

Summary and Discussion

This chapter examined the socio-demographic and psychosocial correlates of continuation or discontinuation of drug use in a sample of young and active or former drug users interviewed at six time points at 6-month intervals for a longitudinal survey of psychoactive drug abusers in Hong Kong conducted from 2009 to 2012. None of the socio-demographic variables was significantly related to drug use in the last 30 days at four or more of the six time points. According to the "normalization of recreational drug use" thesis described in Chap. 1, this was not surprising, as socio-demographic backgrounds were not good predictors of the initiation and continuous consumption of recreational drug use among young people nowadays (Parker et al. 1998; Cheung and Cheung 2006).

On the contrary, continuation/discontinuation of drug use was significantly related to quite a number of psychosocial variables at four or more time points. Results from random-effects probit regression analysis showed that the attitudinal variable of permissiveness to occasional drug use had exerted the greatest influence on drug use in the last 30 days, followed by life satisfaction, permissiveness to regular drug use, and depression. Drug use was also affected by drug use at the previous time point (−1) as well as self-esteem at the previous time point (−1). Self-esteem, however, did not directly affect drug use at the same time point.

As the close link between attitude and behaviour has been well ascertained in social science, the present finding that the two prodrug attitudes significantly affected continuous drug use is not surprising. It is, however, interesting to note that in this study, the effect of permissiveness to occasional drug use on drug use in the last 30 days was greater than that of permissiveness to regular drug use. Again, we think this can be explained by the perspective of normalization of recreational drug use. As a coping mechanism to strong competition and harsh reality faced by young people today, more and more of them, regardless of age, sex, and socioeconomic backgrounds, like going to parties/clubs and consume psychoactive drugs for the temporary pursuit of security, warm feeling, and youth identity. Recreational drug use has become increasingly acceptable to them in both attitude and behaviour. In Hong Kong, prodrug attitude and drug use among young people have been facilitated by a process of "neutralization" of ketamine use (see discussion in Chap. 1), in which (1) ketamine was perceived as a so-called "soft" drug, which, unlike "hard" drugs such as heroin, was much less addictive and much easier to quit if necessary, and (2) ketamine use was considered to be only a "bad habit" rather than a drug addiction, and so as long as they avoid doing heroin, they are safe (Cheung 2015). It is, therefore, not surprising that, among the subjects in this study, a permissive attitude towards *recreational* drug use was even a stronger predictor for continuous drug use than a permissive attitude towards *regular* use. It should be noted, however, that this study did not allow us to further examine if permissiveness to occasional drug use would later bring about higher levels and frequencies of use over time, as data on the frequency and amount of use were not collected.

Life satisfaction and depression also significantly affected continuous drug use. Subjects who were less satisfied with life were more likely to have used a drug in the last 30 days. This echoed the finding of a negative relationship between life satisfaction or psychological well-being and high-risk behaviour in many overseas and local studies (e.g. Bogart et al. 2007; Cheung 2009; Shek 1997, 2002, 2003; Sun and Shek 2010, 2012; Valois et al. 2004; Zullig et al. 2001). As to depression, it was significantly, though only weakly, related to drug use in the last 30 days. Subjects with a higher level of depression were more likely to have used drugs in the last 30 days. This was consistent with the finding of a positive relationship between depression and substance use in adolescents in many studies (e.g. Wu et al. 2008).

We also examined how the two permissive attitude variables as well as other psychosocial variables had affected each other. We conducted a series of regressions, each using a psychosocial variable as the outcome variable and other ones as independent variables.

First, we asked: what were the psychosocial factors that might affect the two kinds of permissive attitudes? Results showed that thinking that doing extreme things shows the vitality of young people was significant in the regressions of both attitudes. The stronger this adventurous belief, the more the permissiveness to regular and occasional drug use. Subjects who wished to have a normal life in future were less likely to be permissive to regular drug use, indicating that some kind of risk assessment might be involved. Those who believed that schools do not know how to teach students were more likely to be permissive to occasional drug use, possibly as an expression of a counter-subculture against the school.

Life satisfaction and self-esteem had also significantly and negatively affected permissiveness to both regular and occasional drug use. At the same time point, the higher the level of life satisfaction, and the higher the self-esteem, the lower the levels of permissiveness to regular and occasional drug use. In addition, the levels of permissive attitudes were affected by self-esteem at the previous time point (−1). Thus, boosting up the self-esteem of the drug user would help to mitigate his/her prodrug attitudes. Not surprisingly, the two permissiveness attitudes were each affected by itself at the previous time point. Thus, prodrug attitudes are quite stable over time. If efforts are not made to successfully reduce it, then prodrug attitudes will remain an obstacle to the discontinuation of drug use. As the effect of permissiveness to occasional drug use at the previous time point on this attitude at the concurrent time point was much greater than that of permissiveness to regular drug use, it was a greater challenge for intervention work to change the permissive attitude towards occasional drug use than towards regular drug use. Lastly, drug use at the previous time point (−1) was a robust variable positively affecting the two permissive attitudes.

Nest, we examined what socio-demographic and psychosocial variables were significantly related to life satisfaction. While permissiveness to occasional drug use, ever been discriminated by other people, and uncertainty about the future at the concurrent time point were significant, their respective beta coefficients were small, suggesting that their predictive powers were not strong for life satisfaction. Stronger beta coefficients were found to come from self-esteem and depression. A higher self-esteem and a lower level of depression could contribute to a higher level of life satisfaction. Life satisfaction at the previous time point (−1) also affected life satisfaction at the current time point, showing that this variable was quite stable over time. Depression (−1) and stricken by stressful events (−1) also affected life satisfaction at the concurrent time point, although their coefficients were much smaller than that of life satisfaction (−1).

We have shown that self-esteem had significant relationships with most of the other psychosocial variables at the current time point as well as the next time point. What psychosocial variables were significantly related to self-esteem? A large number of them at the concurrent time points were. Permissiveness to regular drug use, disappointed if aspired education level is not achieved, sense of uncertainty about future, and depression were negatively related to self-esteem. Life satisfaction, as expected, was positively related. At the previous time point, self-esteem (−1) strongly affected self-esteem at current time point. Depression (−1) and stricken by stressful events (−1) were also significantly, albeit weakly, related to self-esteem.

Lastly, for depression, at concurrent time point, ever been discriminated by other people, sense of uncertainty about future, think that parents don't know how to teach children, and stricken by stressful events were factors significantly, though weakly, contributing to a higher level of depression. Life satisfaction and self-esteem were protective factors against depression. As to effects coming from the previous time point, depression (−1) strongly affected depression at the current time point, as did self-esteem (−1).

References

Bogart, L. M., Collins, R. L., Ellickson, P. L., & Klein, D. J. (2007). Are adolescent substance users less satisfied with life as young adults and if so, why? *Social Indicators Research, 81*, 149–169.

Cheung, Y. W. (2009). *A brighter side: Protective and risk factors in the rehabilitation of chronic drug abusers in Hong Kong*. Hong Kong: The Chinese University Press.

Cheung, Y. W. (2015). Macro social flaws and intervention's unfinished business: A personal note on young people's drug use in Hong Kong. *Substance Use & Misuse, 50*, 1044–1050.

Cheung, N. W. T., & Cheung, Y. W. (2006). Is Hong Kong experiencing normalization of adolescent drug use? Some reflections on the normalization thesis. *Substance Use & Misuse, 41*(14), 1967–1990.

Cheung, N. W. T., Cheung, Y. W., & Chen, X. (2016). Permissive attitude towards drug use, life satisfaction, and continuous drug use among psychoactive drug users in Hong Kong. *East Asian Archives of Psychiatry, 26*, 60–69.

Parker, H., Aldridge, J., & Measham, F. (1998). *Illegal leisure: The normalization of adolescent recreational drug use*. London: Routledge.

Shek, D. T. L. (1997). Family environment and adolescent psychological well-being, school adjustment, and problem behavior: A pioneer study in a Chinese context. *Journal of Genetic Psychology, 158*(1), 113–128.

Shek, D. T. L. (2002). Family environment and psychological well-being, school adjustment, and problem behavior in Chinese adolescents with and without economic disadvantage. *Journal of Genetic Psychology, 163*(4), 497–502.

Shek, D. T. L. (2003). Economic stress, psychological well-being and problem behavior in Chinese adolescents with economic disadvantage. *Journal of Youth and Adolescence, 32*(4), 259–266.

Sun, R. C. F., & Shek, D. T. L. (2010). Life satisfaction, positive youth development, and problem behavior among Chinese adolescents in Hong Kong. *Social Indicators Research, 95*, 455–474.

Sun, R. C. F., & Shek, D. T. L. (2012). Positive youth development, life satisfaction and problem behavior among Chinese adolescents in Hong Kong: A replication. *Social Indicators Research, 105*, 541–559.

Valois, R. F., Zullig, K. J., Huebner, E. S., & Drane, J. W. (2004). Life satisfaction and suicide among high school adolescents. *Social Indicators Research, 66*, 81–105.

Wu, P., Hoven, C., Okezie, N., Fuller, C., & Cohen, P. (2008). Alcohol abuse and depression in children and adolescents. *Journal of Child and Adolescent Substance Abuse, 17*, 51–69.

Zullig, K. J., Valois, R. F., Huebner, E. S., Oeltmann, J. E., & Drane, J. W. (2001). Relationship between perceived life satisfaction and adolescents' substance abuse. *Journal of Adolescent Health, 29*, 279–288.

Chapter 4
Gender Differences in Psychosocial Correlates of Drug Use

The growing convergence of male and female in delinquent involvement is one of the most popular topics in deviance research in recent decades. Several perspectives have been proposed to explain the convergence in relation to social change. Some scholars (e.g. Adler and Adler 1975; Simon 1975) have pointed out that industrialization and modernization have brought about tremendous changes in the life pattern of female—greater participation in the work force, greater opportunity to receive higher or professional education, more gender equality, and being more ready to engage in a broader social life. Liberated from the traditional gender role, women nowadays have more opportunities to commit offences that are formerly much more committed by male. Other scholars doubted the real success of women's movements in achieving gender equality, as male dominance is still prevalent in society. Women's increasing participation in the job market has pushed them into the double role of having to take care of the family and having to work and subject to exploitation in the workplace. This produces great stress in women, who now have greater tendency to turn to drug use or other delinquent behaviours as a coping mechanism (e.g. Chesney-Lind 1989, 1997; Watkins et al. 1994). A third approach is the normalization perspective (Parker et al. 1998; Aldridge et al. 2011) discussed earlier. The growing acceptance and practice of recreational drug use in young people cut across gender and class groups, because through recreational drug use, each group can not only use drugs to cope with tough reality but also create an identity pertinent to their own gender or class backgrounds (Joe Laidler 2005; Measham 2002; Measham et al. 2011).

In Hong Kong, Ng (2012) has conducted an in-depth study of changes in the gender gap in drug use from 1986 to 2009, using police arrest data as well as data from the Central Registry of Drug Abuse, supplemented with results of six self-report student surveys commissioned by the Narcotics Division. Based on the Central Registry of Drug Abuse, for example, the percentage of female drug abusers among all reported drug abusers under age 21 (female percentage, hereafter) grew steadily over the 1990s (from 18% in 1986 to 23% in 1990 and 25% in 1999) and the 2000s (from 28% in 2000 to 31% in 2010) (Lee et al. 2012). The female

Y.W. Cheung, N.W.-t. Cheung, *Psychoactive Drug Abuse in Hong Kong*,
Quality of Life in Asia 11, DOI 10.1007/978-981-10-6154-7_4

percentage remained at 27% in 2015 (Narcotics Division 2016). Ng (2012) concluded that, overall, there was a narrowing of gender gap in drug abuse since the 1980s, and the increase of female drug abuse echoed the perspective that attributes women's drug abuse to the rising levels of stress resulting from the double role that they were caught in. He also remarked that the normalization explanation is pertinent in Hong Kong, as recreational drug use has become more and more acceptable in young people, forming part of the new drug use subculture in them.

The present study targetted drug users and examined whether differences in gender and other socio-demographic characteristics would affect the continuation/discontinuation of drug use of a sample of known drug users. In the last chapter, socio-demographic variables were found to be poor predictors of continuation/discontinuation of drug use, somewhat indirectly supporting the normalization thesis. None of the socio-demographic variables had a significant bivariate relationship with drug use in the last 30 days at four or more time points out of the total of six time points. However, when regressions were performed for the psychosocial variables as outcome variables, gender was able to be bivariately significant at four or more time points with permissiveness to regular drug use, permissiveness to occasional drug use, self-esteem, and depression. Only life satisfaction was not significantly related to gender at four or more time points. If gender was correlated with a lot of psychosocial variables, and since psychosocial variables had effects on the continuation/discontinuation of drug use, we next break the sample into male and female groups and examine and compare the relationships among psychosocial variables and drug use in the two gender groups.

We first compared gender differences in how drug use in the last 30 days was affected by the psychosocial variables and then examined how the psychosocial variables affected each other. As before, the independent variables chosen to be included in the probit regressions were those that had a significant bivariate relationship with the dependent variable at four or more time points. Independent variables included all the psychosocial variables used in the study. In addition, the number of years of drug use was also included for bivariate correlations, as the effects of drug use history would have implications for prevention and intervention efforts. Results of the bivariate relationships between each of the outcome variables and its independent variables for the two gender groups are presented in Appendix Two.

Gender Differences in How Psychosocial Variables Affected Drug Use in the Last 30 Days

In each of following tables showing gender differences in the continuation/discontinuation of drug use as well as psychosocial variables, Model 1was not reported, as it only showed the regression results of variables at the concurrent time point. Model 2 contained effects of variables at both the concurrent and previous time points, and so it would be presented for the comparison of regression results of males and females. Table 4.1 shows the gender differences in drug use in the last 30 days.

Table 4.1 Random-effects probit models of drug use in the last 30 days among males and females on selected psychosocial variables based on data pooled from T2 to T6

	Male		Female	
	Model 2 (N = 1151)		Model 2 (N = 732)	
Independent variables	β	S.E.	β	S.E.
T3	0.129	(0.132)	−0.326	(0.180)
T4	0.166	(0.148)	−0.111	(0.194)
T5	0.042	(0.160)	−0.430*	(0.212)
T6	0.230	(0.172)	−0.482*	(0.233)
Concurrent time point				
Permissiveness to regular drug use	0.184**	(0.062)	0.155	(0.088)
Permissiveness to occasional drug use	0.391***	(0.078)	0.524***	(0.113)
Think that doing extreme things shows the vitality of young people	−0.028	(0.059)	−0.004	(0.086)
Life satisfaction	−0.368***	(0.063)	−0.314***	(0.089)
Self-esteem	−0.100	(0.080)	0.040	(0.108)
Depression	0.081	(0.073)	0.305**	(0.101)
Previous time point				
Drug use in the last 30 days	0.517***	(0.066)	0.404***	(0.091)
Permissiveness to regular drug use	0.012	(0.059)	−0.015	(0.087)
Permissiveness to occasional drug use	−0.009	(0.074)	−0.116	(0.107)
Think that doing extreme things shows the vitality of young people	0.014	(0.055)	0.022	(0.086)
Life satisfaction	−0.003	(0.062)	−0.019	(0.086)
Self-esteem	−0.206**	(0.075)	0.030	(0.100)
Depression	0.080	(0.070)	−0.019	(0.098)
Log likelihood	−482.99		-335.28	
Wald chi-square	281.07***		137.03***	
df	17		17	
Rho	0.14		0.40***	

*$p < .05$; **$p < .01$; ***$p < .001$

All βs are standardized probit coefficients

Rho is the proportion of the total variance explained by the panel-level variance. The significance of Rho means that there is enough variability between individuals to favour a random-effects probit regression (a panel estimator) over a standard probit regression (a pooled estimator)

Only Model 2 of each regression is reported, as Model 1 (as shown in regressions for the whole sample) does not contain results pertaining to previous time point

At the concurrent time point, permissiveness to regular drug use ($\beta = .184$, $p < .01$) and occasional drug use ($\beta = .391$, $p < .001$) were significantly and positively related to drug use in the last 30 days for males, but in females, permissiveness to occasional drug use ($\beta = .524$, $p < .001$) was significant, rather than permissiveness to regular drug use. Life satisfaction negatively affected continuous drug use in both males and females, with similar strengths of effects ($\beta = -.368$, $p < .001$ for males and $\beta = -.314$, $p < .001$ for females). Depression positively affected drug use of females ($\beta = .305$, $p < .01$) but not males. At the previous time point, drug use in the last 30 days (−1) strongly and significantly affected drug use at the concurrent time point for both gender groups ($\beta = .517, p < .001$ for males and $\beta = .404, p < .001$ for females). All psychosocial variables at the previous time point did not affect drug use in the last 30 days at the concurrent time point for both males and females, except self-esteem (−1), which was significantly and negatively associated with drug use for males ($\beta = -.206, p < .01$) only.

From the above results, we can see that although gender was not a good predictor of drug use in the last 30 days, as it yielded a significant bivariate relationship with drug use at only one of the six time points (see Table 3.1), there were both similarities and differences in how psychosocial variables affected drug use in the last 30 days in the two gender groups. As the value of Rho in the regression model for males was not statistically significant, possibly due to small gender-specific panel samples, regression results pertaining to this model should be interpreted with caution.

Gender Differences in How Psychosocial Variables Affected Permissiveness to Regular Drug Use

Both similarities and differences in the contribution of psychosocial variables to permissiveness to regular drug use by gender were detected (Table 4.2).

Among males, three psychosocial variables at the concurrent time point significantly affected permissiveness to regular drug use. Those who held the view that doing extreme things shows the vitality of young people were more likely to accept regular drug ($\beta = .376, p < .001$); those who wished to have own family, job, and normal life in future were less likely to accept regular drug use ($\beta = -.093, p < .05$); and those with a higher level of life satisfaction were less likely to accept regular drug use ($\beta = -.155, p < .001$). Meanwhile, among females, two psychosocial variables at the concurrent time point yielded significant associations with permissiveness to regular drug use. Those females who "think that doing extreme things shows the vitality of young people" were more likely to perceive regular drug use acceptable ($\beta = .291, p < .001$); and those with stronger self-esteem were less likely to accept regular drug use ($\beta = -.223, p < .01$).

Two independent variables at the previous time point had effects on permissiveness to regular drug use among females. They were drug use in the last 30 days (−1) ($\beta = .422, p < .001$) and think that doing extreme things shows the vitality of young people ($\beta = .136, p < .05$). These two variables at the previous time point also affected permissiveness to regular use in males ($\beta = .499, p < .001$ for drug use in the last 30 days (−1); $\beta = .112, p < .01$ for think that doing extreme things shows the vitality of young people). In addition, permissiveness to regular drug use (−1) at the previous time point affected permissiveness to regular drug use at the concurrent time point for males ($\beta = .091, p < .05$) but not females. Taken together, the risk-taking mentality appeared to be a robust predictor for both genders' permissiveness to regular drug use across time points, but life satisfaction and self-esteem contributed differentially to male's and female's attitudes towards regular drug use.

Table 4.2 Random-effects ordered probit models of permissiveness to regular drug use among males and females on selected psychosocial variables based on data pooled from T2 to T6

	Male		Female	
	Model 2 ($N = 1167$)		Model 2 ($N = 735$)	
Independent variables	β	S.E.	β	S.E.
T3	−0.051	(0.095)	−0.017	(0.127)
T4	−0.228*	(0.106)	−0.243	(0.136)
T5	−0.348**	(0.112)	−0.464**	(0.142)
T6	−0.392**	(0.121)	−0.736***	(0.154)
Concurrent time point				
Think that doing extreme things shows the vitality of young people	0.376***	(0.046)	0.291***	(0.062)
Wish to have own family, job, and normal life in future	−0.093*	(0.042)		
Life satisfaction	−0.155***	(0.046)		
Self-esteem			−0.223**	(0.076)
Depression			0.099	(0.069)
Previous time point				
Drug use in the last 30 days	0.499***	(0.094)	0.422***	(0.119)
Permissiveness to regular drug use	0.091*	(0.044)	0.104	(0.060)
Think that doing extreme things shows the vitality of young people	0.112**	(0.042)	0.136*	(0.060)
Wish to have own family, job, and normal life in future	0.043	(0.043)		
Life satisfaction	−0.019	(0.046)		
Self-esteem			0.106	(0.072)
Depression			−0.081	(0.070)
Log likelihood	−1619.30		−974.88	
Wald chi-square	214.15***		133.33***	
df	12		12	
Panel-level variance	1.02***		0.97***	

*$p < .05$; **$p < .01$; ***$p < .001$
All βs are standardized ordered probit coefficients
The significance of the panel-level variance means that there is sufficient variability between individuals to favour a random-effects ordered probit regression (a panel estimator) over a standard ordered probit regression (a pooled estimator)
Only Model 2 of each regression is reported, as Model 1 (as shown in regressions for the whole sample) does not contain results pertaining to previous time point

Gender Differences in How Psychosocial Variables Affected Permissiveness to Occasional Drug Use

Would the predictors of attitude towards regular drug use be able to also predict attitude towards occasional drug use in accounting for gender disparities? Table 4.3 shows contrasting results, however.

At the concurrent time point, three of the psychosocial variables significantly affected male's permissiveness to occasional drug use, namely, "think that doing

Table 4.3 Random-effects ordered probit models of permissiveness to occasional drug use among males and females on selected psychosocial variables and drug use history based on data pooled from T2 to T6

	Male		Female	
	Model 2 (*N* = 1037)		Model 2 (*N* = 737)	
Independent variables	β	S.E.	β	S.E.
T3	0.002	(0.091)	0.085	(0.119)
T4	−0.071	(0.115)	−0.035	(0.126)
T5	−0.120	(0.122)	−0.140	(0.134)
T6	−0.119	(0.117)	−0.277	(0.148)
Concurrent time point				
No. of years of drug use	−0.027	(0.040)		
Think that doing extreme things shows the vitality of young people	0.300***	(0.045)	0.344***	(0.053)
Wish to have own family, job, and normal life in future	−0.059	(0.039)		
Think that parents don't know how to teach children	0.058	(0.044)		
Think that school doesn't know how to teach students	0.128**	(0.040)		
Life satisfaction	−0.102*	(0.045)		
Depression	0.032	(0.051)		
Previous time point				
Drug use in the last 30 days	0.328***	(0.089)	0.226*	(0.009)
Permissiveness to occasional drug use	0.545***	(0.066)	0.670***	(0.077)
Think that doing extreme things shows the vitality of young people	−0.015	(0.043)	−0.040	(0.057)
Wish to have own family, job, and normal life in future	0.015	(0.040)		
Think that parents don't know how to teach children	0.012	(0.045)		
Think that school doesn't know how to teach students	0.025	(0.039)		
Life satisfaction	0.006	(0.044)		
Depression	−0.079	(0.048)		
Log likelihood	−1421.38		−958.62	
Wald chi-square	374.79***		229.73***	
df	19		8	
Panel-level variance	0.15*		0.16***	

*$p < .05$; **$p < .01$; ***$p < .001$

All βs are standardized ordered probit coefficients

The significance of the panel-level variance means that there is sufficient variability between individuals to favour a random-effects ordered probit regression (a panel estimator) over a standard ordered probit regression (a pooled estimator)

Only Model 2 of each regression is reported, as Model 1 (as shown in regressions for the whole sample) does not contain results pertaining to previous time point extreme things shows the vitality of young people" ($\beta = .300$, $p < .001$), "think that school doesn't know how to teach students" ($\beta = .128$, $p < .01$), and life satisfaction ($\beta = -.102$, $p < .05$). For females, only "think that doing extreme things shows the vitality of young people" was significantly related to attitude towards occasional drug use ($\beta = .344$, $p < .001$). As to the previous time point, both drug use in the last 30 days (−1) and permissiveness to occasional drug use (−1) were significant. Drug use in the last 30 days (−1) yielded a probit regression coefficient of .328 ($p < .001$) for males and .226 ($p < .05$) for females. What is interesting to note is that the effect of permissiveness to occasional drug use (−1) at the previous time point on permissiveness to occasional drug use at the concurrent time point was significant and strong for both gender groups ($\beta = .545$, $p < .001$ for males and $\beta = .670$, $p < .001$ for females). This suggests that the attitude towards occasional drug use was quite stable across time in both gender groups. This was in contrast to the attitude towards regular drug use, as permissiveness to regular drug use (−1) was only weakly related to permissiveness to regular drug use at the concurrent time point for males and not significantly related to permissiveness to regular drug use at the concurrent time point for females (see Table 4.2). Thus, permissiveness to regular drug use was not a good predictor of itself at the next time points.

Gender Differences in How Psychosocial Variables Affected Life Satisfaction

There were both similarities and differences in how psychosocial variables were conducive to life satisfaction of the two gender groups (Table 4.4).

At the concurrent time point, self-esteem and depression significantly affected life satisfaction for both groups. The higher the self-esteem, the higher the life satisfaction ($\beta = .337$, $p < .001$ for males and $\beta = .420$, $p < .001$ for females). Conversely, the higher the level of depression, the lower the life satisfaction ($\beta = -.295$, $p < .001$ for males and $\beta = -.404$, $p < .001$ for females). Sense of uncertainty about future affected males ($\beta = .126$, $p < .01$) but not females. Female's life satisfaction was significantly and negatively affected by stricken by stressful events ($\beta = -.129$, $p < .01$), but male's life satisfaction was not. As to the previous time point, life satisfaction (−1) significantly and positively affected life satisfaction at the concurrent time point ($\beta = .334$, $p < .001$ for males and $\beta = .354$, $p < .001$ for females), suggesting that life satisfaction remained stable and strong across time points. Surprisingly, depression (−1) at the previous time point had a positive effect on life satisfaction at the concurrent time point among females ($\beta = .137$, $p < .05$). However, the coefficient was only barely significant ($p < .05$), and the panel-level variance (.09) for the female model was not statistically significant, suggesting that the regression results should be interpreted with caution.

Table 4.4 Random-effects ordered probit models of life satisfaction among males and females on selected psychosocial variables based on data pooled from T2 to T6

	Male		Female	
	Model 2 (N = 1039)		Model 2 (N = 742)	
Independent variable	β	S.E.	β	S.E.
T3	−0.059	(0.094)	−0.072	(0.122)
T4	−0.142	(0.118)	−0.206	(0.128)
T5	0.027	(0.125)	−0.190	(0.132)
T6	−0.023	(0.118)	−0.178	(0.139)
Concurrent time point				
Permissiveness to regular drug use	−0.086	(0.047)		
Permissiveness to occasional drug use	−0.075	(0.055)		
Sense of uncertainty about future	−0.126**	(0.041)	−0.092	(0.054)
Think that parents don't know how to teach children	−0.079	(0.045)		
Think that school doesn't know how to teach students	−0.050	(0.041)		
Self-esteem	0.337***	(0.059)	0.420***	(0.071)
Depression	−0.295***	(0.058)	−0.404***	(0.065)
Stricken by stressful events			−0.129**	(0.048)
Previous time point				
Drug use in the last 30 days	−0.018	(0.044)	−0.035	(0.047)
Life satisfaction	0.334***	(0.057)	0.354***	(0.078)
Permissiveness to regular drug use	0.037	(0.045)		
Permissiveness to occasional drug use	−0.068	(0.053)		
Sense of uncertainty about future	−0.009	(0.041)	−0.096	(0.053)
Think that parents don't know how to teach children	−0.021	(0.046)		
Think that school doesn't know how to teach students	−0.007	(0.040)		
Self-esteem	−0.040	(0.056)	−0.075	(0.067)
Depression	0.048	(0.055)	0.137*	(0.066)
Stricken by stressful events			0.090	(0.046)
Log likelihood	−123.46		−794.80	
Wald chi-square	332.11***		310.35***	
df	20		14	
Panel-level variance	0.13***		0.09	

*$p < .05$; **$p < .01$; ***$p < .001$

All βs are standardized ordered probit coefficients

The significance of the panel-level variance means that there is sufficient variability between individuals to favour a random-effects ordered probit regression (a panel estimator) over a standard ordered probit regression (a pooled estimator)

Only Model 2 of each regression is reported, as Model 1 (as shown in regressions for the whole sample) does not contain results pertaining to previous time point

Gender Differences in How Psychosocial Variables Affected Self-Esteem

At the concurrent time point, sense of uncertainty about future, life satisfaction, and depression significantly affected self-esteem of both gender groups (Table 4.5).

The higher the sense of uncertainty about future, the lower the self-esteem ($\beta = -.085$, $p < .001$ for males and $\beta = -.172$, $p < .001$ for females). The higher the life satisfaction, the higher the self-esteem ($\beta = .131$, $p < .001$ for males and $\beta = .148$, $p < .001$ for females). The higher the level of depression, the lower the self-esteem ($\beta = -.362$, $p < .001$ for males and $\beta = -.359$, $p < .001$ for females). In addition to these three common psychosocial variables, "wish to have own family, job, and normal life in future" positively affected male's self-esteem ($\beta = .110$, $p < .001$), whereas subjective weathering was negatively and weakly related to males' self-esteem ($\beta = -.086$, $p < .001$). For females, permissiveness to regular drug use significantly and negatively affected their self-esteem ($\beta = -.111$, $p < .001$).

Self-esteem (−1) at the previous time point significantly and strongly affected self-esteem at the concurrent time point for both gender groups ($\beta = .392$, $p < .001$ for males and $\beta = .414$, $p < .001$ for females), indicating that self-esteem was quite stable over time. Lastly, depression (−1) at previous time point affected male's self-esteem ($\beta = .062$, $p < .05$) but not female's.

Gender Differences in How Psychosocial Variables Affected Depression

At the concurrent time point, most of the psychosocial variables in the regression had significant effects on depression for both males and females (Table 4.6).

In the male group, significant psychosocial variables included ever been discriminated by other people ($\beta = .091$, $p < .001$), sense of uncertainty about future ($\beta = .111$, $p < .001$), think that parents don't know how to teach children ($\beta = .056$, $p < .05$), think that school doesn't know how to teach students ($\beta = .043$, $p < .05$), life satisfaction ($\beta = -.130$, $p < .001$), self-esteem ($\beta = -.378$, $p < .001$), and stricken by stressful events ($\beta = .096$, $p < .001$). Psychosocial variables that affected females were sense of uncertainty about future ($\beta = .088$, $p < .05$), life satisfaction ($\beta = -.219$, $p < .001$), self-esteem ($\beta = -.404$, $p < .001$), and stricken by stressful events ($\beta = .109$, $p < .001$).

At the previous time point, psychosocial variables that affected the level of depression of males were self-esteem (−1) ($\beta = .135$, $p < .001$) and depression (−1) ($\beta = .312$, $p < .001$), whereas for females, only depression (−1) affected itself at the concurrent time point ($\beta = .293$, $p < .001$). However, regression results in this Table 4.6 should be interpreted with caution, as the Rho values of the two gender models were not statistically significant.

Table 4.5 Random-effects maximum likelihood linear models of self-esteem among males and females on selected psychosocial variables based on data pooled from T2 to T6

	Male		Female	
	Model 2 (N = 1151)		Model 2 (N = 622)	
Independent variable	β	S.E.	β	S.E.
T3	−0.015	(0.048)	0.019	(0.069)
T4	0.031	(0.053)	−0.012	(0.074)
T5	-0.043	(0.054)	−0.050	(0.075)
T6	0.066	(0.059)	−0.041	(0.082)
Concurrent time point				
Permissiveness to regular drug use			−0.111***	(0.029)
Level of disappointment if aspired education level is not achieved			−0.053	(0.029)
Ever been discriminated by other people	0.018	(0.022)		
Sense of uncertainty about future	−0.085***	(0.019)	−0.172***	(0.031)
Think that doing extreme things shows vitality of young people			−0.051	(0.031)
Wish to have own family, job, and normal life in future	0.110***	(0.019)		
Think that parents don't know how to teach children	−0.031	(0.022)		
Life satisfaction	0.131***	(0.022)	0.148***	(0.031)
Depression	−0.362***	(0.026)	−0.359***	(0.034)
Subjective weathering	−0.086***	(0.023)		
Previous time point				
Drug use in the last 30 days	0.025	(0.020)	0.038	(0.029)
Self-esteem	0.392***	(0.045)	0.414***	(0.065)
Permissiveness to regular drug use			0.037	(0.030)
Level of disappointment if aspired education level is not achieved			0.007	(0.029)
Ever been discriminated by other people	-0.009	(0.021)		
Sense of uncertainty about future	0.026	(0.020)	0.045	(0.032)
Think that doing extreme things shows vitality of young people			0.019	(0.031)
Wish to have own family, job, and normal life in future	−0.036	(0.020)		
Think that parents don't know how to teach children	0.021	(0.022)		
Life satisfaction	0.002	(0.023)	−0.046	(0.033)
Depression	0.062*	(0.029)	0.068	(0.044)
Subjective weathering	0.029	(0.022)		
Log likelihood	−1039.57		−576.80	
Likelihood ratio chi-square	569.55***		420.03***	
df	20		18	
Rho	0.10*		0.12*	

*$p < .05$; **$p < .01$; ***$p < .001$
All βs are standardized coefficients
Rho is the proportion of the total variance explained by the panel-level variance. The significance of Rho means that there is enough variability between individuals to favour a random-effects probit regression (a panel estimator) over a standard probit regression (a pooled estimator)

Table 4.6 Random-effects maximum likelihood linear models of depression among males and females on selected psychosocial variables based on data pooled from T2 toT6

	Male		Female	
	Model 2 ($N = 1034$)		Model 2 ($N = 554$)	
Independent variable	β	S.E.	β	S.E.
T3	−0.012	(0.051)	−0.085	(0.074)
T4	−0.021	(0.064)	0.077	(0.087)
T5	0.004	(0.066)	−0.042	(0.089)
T6	0.015	(0.063)	0.137	(0.087)
Concurrent time point				
Permissiveness to regular drug use			0.031	(0.032)
Permissiveness to occasional drug use	−0.003	(0.025)		
Level of disappointment if aspired education level is not achieved			0.040	(0.032)
Ever been discriminated by other people	0.091***	(0.024)	0.045	(0.035)
Sense of uncertainty about future	0.111***	(0.021)	0.088*	(0.035)
Think that parents don't know how to teach children	0.056*	(0.024)	0.043	(0.036)
Think that school doesn't know how to teach students	0.043*	(0.022)	0.024	(0.031)
Life satisfaction	−0.130***	(0.024)	−0.219***	(0.035)
Self-esteem	−0.378***	(0.029)	−0.404***	(0.042)
Stricken by stressful events	0.096***	(0.022)	0.109***	(0.031)
Previous time point				
Drug use in the last 30 days	0.027	(0.023)	0.028	(0.032)
Permissiveness to regular drug use			0.039	(0.032)
Permissiveness to occasional drug use	0.020	(0.025)		
Level of disappointment if aspired education level is not achieved			0.040	(0.031)
Ever been discriminated by other people	−0.012	(0.023)	−0.009	(0.033)
Sense of uncertainty about future	−0.002	(0.021)	−0.043	(0.034)
Think that parents don't know how to teach children	−0.018	(0.024)	0.022	(0.035)
Think that school doesn't know how to teach students	−0.010	(0.021)	0.058	(0.031)
Life satisfaction	0.046	(0.024)	0.043	(0.036)
Self-esteem	0.135***	(0.031)	0.082	(0.045)
Depression	0.312***	(0.039)	0.293***	(0.057)
Stricken by stressful events	0.013	(0.021)	0.048	(0.030)
Log likelihood	−965.38		−537.60	
Likelihood ratio chi-square	548.38***		415.93***	
df	22		24	
Rho	0.01		0.09	

*$p < .05$; **$p < .01$; ***$p < .001$

All βs are standardized coefficients

Rho is the proportion of the total variance explained by the panel-level variance. The significance of Rho means that there is enough variability between individuals to favour a random-effects probit regression (a panel estimator) over a standard probit regression (a pooled estimator)

Gender Differences: A Summary

The above-mentioned results pertaining to gender differences in how psychosocial variables had affected drug use in the last 30 days and how they had affected each other can be summarized in Table 4.7.

Table 4.7 clearly shows that there were both similarities and differences in the two gender groups. When drug use in the last 30 days was the outcome variable, permissiveness to occasional drug use and life satisfaction at the concurrent time point, as well as drug use in the last 30 days (−1) at the previous time point, were significant for males and females, whereas permissiveness to regular drug use and self-esteem (−1) were significant only for males, and depression was significant for females only.

When permissiveness to regular drug use was the outcome variable, psychosocial variables had much more significant effects in the male group than in the female group. When permissiveness to occasional drug use was the outcome variable, the view that doing extreme things shows the vitality of young people had affected both males and females. When it comes to life satisfaction, both groups were affected by self-esteem and depression as well as life satisfaction (−1). But there were also differences: males' life satisfaction was affected by sense of uncertainty about future, and females' life satisfaction was affected by stricken by stressful events. For self-esteem, sense of uncertainty about future, life satisfaction, and depression had affected the self-esteem of both males and females. Males' self-esteem was also affected by the wish to have own family, job, and normal life in future, subjective weathering, and depression (−1); whereas females' self-esteem was affected by their permissiveness to regular drug use and self-esteem (−1). In the case of depression, common significant psychosocial variables included sense of uncertainty about future, life satisfaction, self-esteem, and stricken by stressful events at concurrent time point and depression (−1) at previous time point. But there were variables that only affected males but not females, which included ever been discriminated by other people, think that parents don't know how to teach children, and think that school doesn't know how to teach students.

Discussion

The first most striking result on the gender dimension in this chapter relates to the permissiveness to the two different modes of psychoactive drug use. We observed a much stronger impact of the receptive attitude towards occasional drug use for females' than males' drug taking behaviour. Also, females' receptive attitude towards occasional use was a stable predictor of its value at subsequent time points, but their attitude towards regular use was not steadfastly stable and subject to change across time points. This pattern, however, was less pronounced in male drug users. Rather, there was clearer stability of permissiveness to regular use in males. These findings tend to support gendered normalization discussed in the

Table 4.7 Summary of gender differences in the relationships between psychosocial variables and drug use in the last 30 days and relationships among psychosocial variables

	Drug use in the last 30 days		Permissiveness to regular drug use		Permissiveness to occasional drug use		Life satisfaction		Self-esteem		Depression	
Independent variables	M	F	M	F	M	F	M	F	M	F	M	F
Concurrent time point												
Permissiveness to regular drug use	+									–		
Permissiveness to occasional drug use	+	+										
Level of disappointment if aspired education level is not achieved												
Ever been discriminated by other people											+	
Sense of uncertainty about future							–		–	–	+	+
Think that doing extreme things shows vitality of young people			+		+	+						
Think that parents don't know how to teach children											+	
Think that school doesn't know how to teach students					+						+	
Wish to have own family, job, and normal life in future			–						+			
Life satisfaction	–	–	–		–				+	+	–	–
Self-esteem							+	+			–	–
Depression		+					–	–	–	–		
Subjective weathering									–			
Stricken by stressful events								–			+	+

(continued)

Table 4.7 (continued)

Independent variables	Drug use in the last 30 days		Permissiveness to regular drug use		Permissiveness to occasional drug use		Life satisfaction		Self-esteem		Depression	
	M	F	M	F	M	F	M	F	M	F	M	F
Previous time point												
Drug use in the last 30 days (−1)	+	+	+	+	+	+						
Permissiveness to regular drug use (−1)			+									
Permissiveness to occasional drug use (−1)					+	+						
Level of disappointment if aspired education level is not achieved												
Ever been discriminated by other people (−1)												
Sense of uncertainty about future (−1)												
Think that doing extreme things shows vitality of young people (−1)			+	+								
Think that parents don't know how to teach children (−1)												
Think that school doesn't know how to teach students (−1)												
Wish to have own family, job, and normal life in future (−1)												
Life satisfaction (−1)							+	+				
Self-esteem (−1)	+									+	+	
Depression (−1)									+		+	+
Subjective weathering (−1)												
Stricken by stressful events (−1)												

drugs field. Although there is more cultural accommodation and practice of recreational drug use across gender as mentioned at the outset of this chapter, we should be sensitive to the meanings of recreational drug use for different genders. Measham's (2002) seminal work on revisiting gender in contemporary drug culture identified that doing gender in normalizing recreational drug culture is achieved in the overlapping recreational spheres of men's and women's accomplishment of both masculinities and femininities through their drug consumption. One typical example concerns the gendered expectation of drugs: young men tend to relate high intoxication from club drugs to street masculinity, whereas girls are more likely to exercise self-control and minimize intoxication/loss of control so as to enact norms of feminine conformity. Drug use marked by personal agency allows women to escape from passive femininity (Ettorre 2004). That is why there was greater preference over occasional use in females, but not males, as found in the present study.

Furthermore, notions of consumption as mundane, pleasurable, and fitting into everyday lives, rather than causing dependency and misery, are evident not only in today's male drug users but also their female peers (Measham 2002; Measham et al. 2011), who have moved away from their traditional portrayals as double-marginalized drug addicts (being a deviant and a female role violator) and victims discriminated against in the primarily male-dominated illicit drug market (Ettorre 2004; Maher 1997). Our results also seem to align with those notions that the risk-taking mentality (measured by an indicator that doing extreme things shows the vitality of young people), instead of depression and stressful life experiences, was found to play a role in enhancing the permissiveness to occasional drug use among young females. This kind of evidence implies that drug use is not necessarily a miserable experience for our female subsample. In short, our study suggests that gendered normalization likely prevails in the Chinese setting as well. Because measures of gender beliefs were not available in this study, further investigation of gender norms concerning recreational versus regular use of psychoactive drugs in the Chinese context is warranted.

Second, the understanding of gender and psychoactive drug use should be sensitive to the positive psychological development in relation to life satisfaction. The stability of life satisfaction across time points and as a proximate factor useful for reduction of drug use behaviour was found to be present in both genders. Still, some gender differences are noteworthy: life satisfaction more stably predicted both drug use behaviour and attitudes for male drug users, indicating that males who are more satisfied with life are less likely to use drugs and maintain prodrug attitudes. It may be the case that men usually score higher on life satisfaction than women (Donohue et al. 2003; Kwan 2010; Moksnes and Espnes 2013), and accordingly men may have more psychological resources to cope with drug-taking propensity. While the finding underscores the greater importance of life satisfaction for male psychoactive drug users, more broadly it adds to the literature on life satisfaction and drug use that seldom addresses gender differences (e.g. Bogart et al. 2007; Maeyer et al. 2009; Sun and Shek 2010, 2012). One exception was the study of whites and blacks conducted by Zullig et al. (2001), who showed gender variations in the relationship between life satisfaction and use of drugs to be modest. Given the salience of life satisfaction and as further suggested by our results, increasing self-esteem, overcoming depression, and mitigating sense of uncertainty about future are key to the enhancement of life satisfaction for male drug users.

The third major issue that emerged from our gender analyses is the notable role of depression in females' psychoactive drug use but not in male's drug use. Female users who were depressed tended to persist in taking psychoactive drugs. Depression, in conjunction with exposure to stressful life events, was also found to link to lower life satisfaction of female drug users, which was a proximate factor associated with their drug use pinpointed earlier. While the relationship between depression and life satisfaction was likely to be recursive, our results tended to evince a stronger influence of depression on life satisfaction, rather than the other way round. Higher vulnerability to depression and stressful life experiences among female users relative to their male peers may be attributed to gender role identifications. Marcotte et al. (1999) have argued that when youth develop gender role identifications, males become more prone to develop instrumental characteristics that act as protective mechanisms against depressive symptoms. At the same time, females become less confident in their problem-solving capabilities, whereas the opposite exists among males. The gender role identifications and concomitant differences in coping strategies may explain why young females react more severely to stress in the form of self-directed negative affect (depression or anxiety) (Abada et al. 2008; Broidy and Agnew 1997; Jang 2007; Kaufman 2009), which in turn is conducive to their substance abuse behaviour (De Coster and Zito 2010; Francis 2014).

References

Abada, T., Hou, F., & Ram, B. (2008). The effects of harassment and victimization on self-rated health and mental health among Canadian adolescents. *Social Science & Medicine, 67*, 557–567.

Adler, F., & Adler, H. M. (1975). *Sisters in crime: The rise of the new female criminal*. New York: McGraw Hill.

Aldridge, J., Measham, F., & Willams, L. (2011). *Illegal leisure revisited: Changing patterns of alcohol and drug use in adolescents and young adults*. New York: Routledge.

Bogart, L. M., Collins, R. L., Ellickson, P. L., & Klein, D. J. (2007). Are adolescent substance users less satisfied with life as young adults and if so, why? *Social Indicators Research, 81*, 149–169.

Broidy, L., & Agnew, R. (1997). Gender and crime: A general strain theory approach. *Journal of Research in Crime and Delinquency, 34*, 275–306.

Chesney-Lind, M. (1989). Girls' crime and woman's place: Toward a feminist model of female delinquency. *Crime & Delinquency, 35*, 5–29.

Chesney-Lind, M. (1997). *The female offender: Girls, women, and crime*. Thousand Oaks: Sage Publications.

De Coster, S., & Zito, R. C. (2010). Gender and general strain theory: The gendering of emotional experiences and expressions. *Journal of Contemporary Criminal Justice, 26*, 224–245.

Donohue, B., Teichner, G., Azrin, N., Weintraub, N., Crum, T. A., Murphy, L., & Sliver, N. C. (2003). Initial reliability and validity of the life satisfaction scale for problem youth in a sample of drug using and conduct disordered youth. *Journal of Child and Family Studies, 12*, 453–464.

Ettorre, E. (2004). Revisioning women and drug use: Gender sensitivity, embodiment and reducing harm. *International Journal of Drug Policy, 15*, 327–335.

Francis, K. A. (2014). General strain theory, gender, and the conditioning influence of negative internalizing emotions on youth risk behaviors. *Youth Violence and Juvenile Justice, 12*, 58–76.

Jang, S. J. (2007). Gender differences in strain, negative emotions, and coping behaviors: A general strain theory approach. *Justice Quarterly, 24*, 523–533.

Joe Laidler, K. A. (2005). The rise of club drugs in a heroin society: The case of Hong Kong. *Substance Use & Misuse, 40*, 1257–1278.

Kaufman, J. M. (2009). Gendered responses to serious strain: The argument for a general strain theory of deviance. *Justice Quarterly, 26*, 410–444.

Kwan, Y. K. (2010). Life satisfaction and self-assessed health among adolescents in Hong Kong. *Journal of Happiness Studies, 11*, 383–393.

Lee, K. W. K., Cheung, N. W. T., & Zhong, S. H. (2012). Victimization and risk behaviors among girl-child in Hong Kong. In S. Y. P. Choi & F. M. Cheung (Eds.), *Women and girls in Hong Kong: Current situations and future challenges* (pp. 265–294). Hong Kong: Hong Kong Institute of Asia-Pacific Studies, The Chinese University of Hong Kong.

Maeyer, J. D., Vanderplasschen, W., & Broekaert, E. (2009). Exploratory study on drug users' perspectives on quality of life: More than health-related quality of life? *Social Indicators Research, 90*, 107–126.

Maher, L. (1997). *Sexed work: Gender, race, and resistance in a Brooklyn drug market*. Oxford: Clarendon.

Marcotte, D., Alain, M., & Gosselin, M. J. (1999). Gender differences in adolescent depression: Gender-types characteristics or problem-solving skills deficits? *Sex Roles, 41*, 31–48.

Measham, F. (2002). 'Doing gender' – 'Doing drugs': Conceptualizing the gendering of drugs cultures. *Contemporary Drug Problems, 29*, 335–373.

Measham, F., Williams, L., & Aldridge, J. (2011). Marriage, mortgage and motherhood: What longitudinal studies can tell us about gender, drug 'careers' and the normalisation of adult 'recreational' drug use. *International Journal of Drug Policy, 22*, 420–427.

Moksnes, U. K., & Espnes, G. A. (2013). Self-esteem and life satisfaction in adolescents – Gender and age as potential moderators. *Quality of Life Research, 22*, 2921–2928.

Narcotics Division. (2016). *Central registry of drug abuse sixty-fifth report (2006-2015)*. Hong Kong: Narcotics Division, Security Bureau, Government of the Hong Kong SAR.

Ng, D.K.S. (2012). *Explaining gender gap in illicit drug use: Evidence from a time-series analysis*. Ph.D. thesis, Department of Sociology, The Chinese University of Hong Kong.

Parker, H., Aldridge, J., & Measham, F. (1998). *Illegal leisure: The normalization of adolescent recreational drug use*. London: Routledge.

Simon, R. J. (1975). *Women and crime*. Lexington: Lexington Books.

Sun, R. C. F., & Shek, D. T. L. (2010). Life satisfaction, positive youth development, and problem behavior among Chinese adolescents in Hong Kong. *Social Indicators Research, 95*, 455–474.

Sun, R. C. F., & Shek, D. T. L. (2012). Positive youth development, life satisfaction and problem behavior among Chinese adolescents in Hong Kong: A replication. *Social Indicators Research, 105*, 541–559.

Watkins, S. A., Rueda, M., & Rodriguez, M. (1994). *Introducing feminism*. Duxford: Icon Books.

Zullig, K. J., Valois, R. F., Huebner, E. S., Oeltmann, J. E., & Drane, J. W. (2001). Relationship between perceived life satisfaction and adolescents' substance abuse. *Journal of Adolescent Health, 29*, 279–288.

Chapter 5
Probing into the Role of Subjective Well-Being in the Rehabilitation of Psychoactive Drug Abusers

In Chap. 3, the influence of socio-demographic factors and psychosocial factors in psychoactive drug use was examined. It was found that none of the socio-demographic variables was significantly related to drug use in the last 30 days at four or more of the six time points (Table 3.1). Thus, socio-demographic variables were not good predictors of the continuation or discontinuation of drug use. On the contrary, a large number of psychosocial variables were found to be significant at four or more time points. They were selected for multivariate analyses using the probit regression method. The results showed that four of these psychosocial variables remained significant, namely, permissiveness to regular drug use, permissiveness to occasional drug use, life satisfaction, and depression (Table 3.3). Self-esteem at the previous time point affected drug use at the concurrent time point, but self-esteem at the concurrent time point did not. The significance of these variables on drug use in the last 30 days was present in both gender groups, although there were some differences between the male and female groups in the effects of these psychosocial variables on drug use in the last 30 days.

In this chapter, we focus on two of the above-mentioned significant psychosocial variables, which are life satisfaction and depression, and discuss their potential roles in the treatment and rehabilitation of psychoactive drug abusers. Life satisfaction is an individual's overall assessment of his/her quality of life, with respect to the extent his/her major needs and goals are fulfilled. It is regarded as a key construct of the broader concept of "subjective well-being" (e.g. Cummins 2003; Diener and Diener 1995). A person who is satisfied with his/her life is someone who has a high degree of subjective well-being. If subjective well-being is a psychological state resulting from the satisfaction with life, then a condition of depression undermines the satisfaction of life and contributes to the lowering of subjective well-being. Here, subjective well-being is meant to include both life satisfaction and depression. We will discuss how the findings in this study pertaining to life satisfaction and depression may be relevant to drug treatment and rehabilitation.

Y.W. Cheung, N.W.-t. Cheung, *Psychoactive Drug Abuse in Hong Kong*, Quality of Life in Asia 11, DOI 10.1007/978-981-10-6154-7_5

Life Satisfaction

Subjective well-being, quality of life, and happiness are frequently researched topics in the social and health sciences. In the past two or three decades, researchers in the field have actively conducted studies of Chinese populations, including Mainland China (e.g. Brockmann et al. 2009; Chen and Davey 2008; Shu and Zhu 2009; Smyth et al. 2010; Ye et al. 2013), Taiwan (e.g. Ip and Cheung 2014; Liao 2009; Tsou and Liu 2001), and Hong Kong (e.g. Lee et al. 1979; Shek 2010; Sing 2009; Wan et al. 2008). Efforts were also made to compare the quality of life in Chinese societies with those in the larger Asian or global contexts (e.g. Inoguchi and Fujii 2013; Shek et al. 2005; Shek and Hollister 2017). While subjective well-being research is flourishing, more research on the quality of life of adolescents needs to be conducted in order to better understand the process of youth development (Shek 2010; Shek and Liu 2014). Existing literature has shown that there is a positive and reciprocal relationship between life satisfaction and youth development (Huebner 2004; Proctor et al. 2009; Shek and Liu 2014). This is particularly relevant to the present study. If among adolescents, a low level of life satisfaction is associated with a higher tendency to be involved in substance abuse (e.g. Bogart et al. 2007; Shek 1997, 2002, 2003; Sun and Shek 2010, 2012; Valois et al. 2004; Zullig et al. 2001), then for the drug users in the present sample, their levels of life satisfaction may affect their continuation or discontinuation of drug use.

Findings of this study confirmed the significant and negative relationship between life satisfaction and continuation of drug use (Chap. 3). Subjects with a higher level of life satisfaction at a time point were more likely to have discontinued drug use at the same time point (Table 3.3). The regression coefficient was strong ($\beta = -.350$, $p < .001$), and in fact, it was only second to the coefficient of permissiveness to occasional drug use ($\beta = .438$, $p < .001$). The significance of the relationship and the strength of the regression coefficients were quite similar in the two gender groups (Table 4.1). An obvious implication of this finding for drug treatment and rehabilitation programmes is the need to raise the level of life satisfaction of the young clients in these programmes.

The strong effect of life satisfaction on drug use is not limited to young drug abusers. Incidentally, the senior author had conducted a 3-year "Longitudinal Study of Chronic Drug Abusers" (primarily heroin abusers) in Hong Kong from 2000 to 2003 (Cheung 2009). Subjects were recruited from various drug treatment and rehabilitation programmes and were interviewed three times at two 1-year intervals. The sample size was 547 subjects at the baseline interview and 401 and 319 in the second and third waves of interviews, respectively. The sample at the third wave of interview (319 subjects, mean age was 36.3) was used for analysis, as these subjects had gone through all three interviews. The dependent variable concerning drug-using or drug-free status was measured by "percentage of drug-free weeks", which referred to the percentage of weeks that the subject was drug-free among the total number of weeks that he/she was not in a residential programme in the interval concerned. Path analysis results showed that, in the same 1-year interval, the total effect (direct and indirect effects) of life satisfaction (.225) on percentage of drug-free weeks was quite similar to that of association with drug-using friends (−.286), although the strongest effect came from self-efficacy (.483).

In the chronic drug abusers study, life satisfaction was measured with a modified version of the scale developed by Diener et al. (1985), which used five items (5-point scale) to assess a subject's overall satisfaction with life (score range was 5–25). The mean of the overall life satisfaction scale was 14.02, 14.37, and 14.21 for the three waves of interviews, respectively. These scores were somewhat below the average score (15.5) of the scale. The sample of young psychoactive drug abusers in the present survey also did not exhibit a high level of life satisfaction. Life satisfaction was measured with a "global approach" making use of one item (5-point scores; 1 = lowest; 5 = highest) that asked the subject to give an overall appraisal of his/her life in general. The mean life satisfaction score ranged from 3.01 to 3.40 for the six time points, indicating only a medium level of life satisfaction. In both studies, life satisfaction was a robust variable that significantly affected drug use in all the intervals or at all the time points.

How Can the Level of Life Satisfaction of Drug Abusers Be Raised?

In the chronic drug abusers study, the senior author pointed out that one of the reasons for the relative low level of satisfaction of chronic drug abusers was relative deprivation (Cheung 2009). Subjects of that study were older adults who had wasted a good chunk of their lives on drug addiction, missing opportunities to build a successful career and raise a normal family. On the contrary, many of the subjects in this study were still in their adolescence, and thus setting up a family and career were still too far fledged to worry. They were more concerned about their immediate lives. It is interesting to note what several male participants of a focus group session comprising Secondary Form 1 to Form 3 students referred by outreach social workers had said about how they could become happier. Quite a few of them suggested that social workers could organize activities that girls would also participate. They liked to meet with girls, especially those from other schools. Such request was understandable, given that these were adolescents in their puberty.

Although most young psychoactive drug users do not have a long view of the future, it does not mean that they will not develop a sense of relative deprivation. Most of the students in our focus group sessions expressed that schooling was very boring. There was a serious lack of motivation to study hard. Very soon they became low achievers in school, gradually developing a deviant subculture in school that de-emphasized mainstream school values and promoted the involvement in risk behaviours. In a way, they had a strong sense of a bleak future because of their poor academic performance. As a Secondary Form 2 student remarked at the focus group meeting:

> I've tried to set higher aspirations for myself before, such as entering the university in future, but it wouldn't be likely for me to achieve that. So, why fancy about it?

Like the case of older and chronic drug abusers, a strong sense of relative deprivation was also an impediment to adolescent drug users' life satisfaction. Organizing activities that young people enjoy will help to make their lives less boring and thus can enhance their life satisfaction. For adolescent drug users who will soon enter young adulthood, they may start to worry about their future. If they are no longer able to go back to school for higher levels of education, then there is the need to help them not to compare with schoolmates with good academic performance but to lower their aspiration in order to minimize frustration and shift their perception of importance in various life domains (Wu 2009).

Besides organizing attractive activities for adolescent drug users and helping them to dilute their feeling of relative deprivation, some clues into the ways to enhance their life satisfaction can be gained by referring to the findings of this study on the psychosocial variables that were significantly related to life satisfaction (Table 3.9). When life satisfaction was the outcome variable in the regression model, significant psychosocial variables at the concurrent time point included:

- Self-esteem ($\beta = .350, p < .001$)
- Depression ($\beta = -.317, p < .001$)
- Permissiveness to occasional drug use ($\beta = -.107, p < .05$)
- Sense of uncertainty about future ($\beta = -.106, p < .01$)
- Ever been discriminated by other people ($\beta = -.073, p < .05$)

Variables at the previous time point that affected life satisfaction at the concurrent time point were:

- Life satisfaction (−1) ($\beta = .369, p < .001$)
- Depression (−1) ($\beta = .090, p < .05$)
- Stricken by stressful events (−1) ($\beta = .073, p < .05$).

From these results, it is obvious that depression and self-esteem were the strongest predictors of life satisfaction. Depression even exerted influence on life satisfaction at two consecutive time points. Thus, at a time point, if the level of depression was reduced, then the likelihood of stopping drug use at the same time point as well as the next time point would increase. Self-esteem at the concurrent time point was as strongly associated with life satisfaction as depression, although self-esteem at the previous time point did not exert any significant effect on life satisfaction. An increase in self-esteem would bring about a greater likelihood of not using any drug at the same time point. These findings serve to inform programmes and services that enhancing self-esteem and reducing depression should be two of the most important elements in their rehabilitation strategies. It should be noted, however, that there were gender differences in how self-esteem and depression affected life satisfaction (Table 4.4). At the same time point, life satisfaction was significantly related to sense of uncertainty about future in the male group but not the female group. Stricken by stressful events significantly influenced female's life satisfaction, but not male's. These gender differences should be taken into account in designing strategies to improve the life satisfaction of young psychoactive drug users.

As mentioned above, in addition to self-esteem and depression, several other psychosocial variables were also significantly related to life satisfaction at the concurrent time point. They were permissiveness to occasional drug use, ever been discriminated by other people, and sense of uncertainty about future. Although these variables yielded very small regression coefficients only, it is nevertheless worthwhile to consider them in rehabilitation strategies in so far as possible.

Life satisfaction at one time point was a strong predictor of life satisfaction at the next time point, and this characteristic was found in both male and female groups. The implication is that if life satisfaction is raised at one time point, then it will very likely enhance life satisfaction at the next time point. By the same token, a low level of life satisfaction at a time point will likely make it harder to raise the level of life satisfaction at the next time point.

Depression

Compared with the two permissive attitudes and life satisfaction, depression yielded a significant, but much smaller, regression coefficient on drug use in the last 30 days ($\beta = .140$, $p < .05$) (Table 3.3). A closer look at the gender groups revealed that depression significantly and strongly ($\beta = .305$, $p < .01$) affected drug use in the last 30 days in females but was not significant among males (Table 4.1). This implies that efforts made to reduce the level of depression of drug users in a treatment and rehabilitation programme would be more effective in stopping drug use of female clients than male clients. Of course, depression is a psychological condition that requires the help of professional counselling services, and such services, if available, should be offered to both female and male clients.

Findings of this study pertaining to psychosocial factors affecting depression can also suggest ways to reduce the level of depression of drug users (Table 4.6). In the female group, at the concurrent time point, psychosocial variables that were significantly associated with depression were:

- Self-esteem ($\beta = -.404$, $p < .001$)
- Life satisfaction ($\beta = -.219$, $p < .001$)
- Stricken by stressful events ($\beta = .109$, $p < .001$)
- Sense of uncertainty about future ($\beta = .088$, $p < .05$).

No variables at the previous time point significantly affected depression, except depression (−1) itself ($\beta = .293$, $p < .001$).

Compared with the female group, there were similarities and differences in the male group. Like in the female group, self-esteem was a significant and the strongest predictor ($\beta = -.378$, $p < .001$) of depression at the concurrent time point among males, followed by life satisfaction ($\beta = -.130$, $p < .001$), sense of uncertainty about future ($\beta = .111$, $p < .001$), and stricken by stressful events ($\beta = .096$,

$p < .001$). Unlike females, males were affected by a few more psychosocial variables, namely, ever been discriminated by other people ($\beta = .091, p < .001$), the view that parents don't know how to teach children ($\beta = .056, p < .05$), and the view that school doesn't know how to teach students ($\beta = .043, p < .05$).

As to the influence of variables at the previous time point, depression (−1) significantly affected itself at the concurrent time point for both genders ($\beta = .293$, $p < .001$ for females and $\beta = .312, p < .001$ for males). Self-esteem (−1) at the previous time point affected depression in males ($\beta = .135, p < .001$) but not females. Overall, self-esteem was the strongest predictor of depression. An improvement in self-esteem will likely bring about a reduction of the level of depression.

Subjective Well-Being as Outcome of Treatment and Rehabilitation

We have examined how life satisfaction and depression affected the continuation or discontinuation of drug use, as well as how other psychosocial variables were significantly related to life satisfaction and depression. We have also suggested that these findings can be incorporated in the improvement of rehabilitation strategies for programmes and services. In the past two decades, as positive psychology began to be popular (Seligman 2002), the potential role of subjective well-being in the drug rehabilitation process has been further explored. A widely explored issue is the incorporation of subjective well-being as one of the treatment outcomes.

In the drug treatment field, the conventional approach focuses predominantly on the termination of drug use as the major outcome as well as its behavioural consequences such as absence of relapse and criminal involvement or recidivism. In recent years, there has been a growing recognition in treatment research on the need to include quality of life in the evaluation of the effectiveness of treatment. Drug abuse worsens quality of life, and so the cessation of drug use should enhance quality of life. Nevertheless, treatments could also bring about iatrogenic effects that could reduce quality of life, even though drug use is stopped or reduced. Therefore, successful treatments should not only help the clients to stop drug use but also enhance their quality of life. In other words, quality of life should be included in treatment and rehabilitation programmes as one of the treatment outcomes (Smith and Larson 2003; Torrens 2008).

But given that quality of life is a very broad concept and has been defined and measured in many ways by researchers, how can a set of criteria for determining this treatment outcome be constructed? One of the attempts was carried out by Maeyer and her colleagues, who considered it necessary to gauge the drug users' perspectives on quality of life, so that the treatment outcome of quality of life should be congruent with the drug users' views and expectations (Maeyer et al. 2009). They conducted nine focus groups in an area in Belgium, comprising drug users of various backgrounds, and analysed the data obtained with the quality of life framework developed by Schalock (1996), which included eight domains, namely, personal relationships, social inclusion, personal development, self-determination, rights, emotional well-being, material well-being, and physical well-being. Data collected from focus group sessions showed that while all the domains were important to the quality of life of drug users, personal relationships, social inclusion, and self-determination were most frequently discussed in the sessions. Good personal relationships, participation in social groups or the community, and opportunities to make decisions in various aspects of life are essential to life in the post-treatment period.

While it is important to take into account the drug users' subjective views of what quality of life should consist of, Tiffany and his colleagues reported on an effort in another approach, which asked experts to make judgements on potential treatment outcomes (Tiffany et al. 2011). In 2009, the National Institute on Drug Abuse (NIDA) in the USA convened a panel of experts on substance abuse treatment and research to review possible outcome measures for clinical trials of drug abuse treatments. Out of 22 potential outcome domains considered by a work group of the panel, which covered drug use and treatment, health, and psychological and social functioning, five domains met the guidelines for inclusion and were recommended as outcomes in treatment. These candidate outcomes were "change self-efficacy", "craving", "psychosocial functioning", "quality of life", and "social network/social support". Tiffany and his colleagues further discussed craving and quality of life as an illustration of how the candidate outcomes can be incorporated into treatment programmes (Tiffany et al. 2011).

Subjective well-being has also been integrated into the Community Reinforcement Approach (CRA), originally developed for treating problematic alcohol use and later employed to treat drug abusers as well (Meyers et al. 2005, 2011). The major objective of CRA is to help people with alcohol or drug problems to modify their lifestyles so that healthy, sober, or drug-free living is experienced to be more rewarding than alcohol or drug use. Drug-free living is reinforced by the drug user's "community", which includes family, work, and friends. The strategy, therefore, is to help the clients to discover new and enjoyable activities that do not involve alcohol or drugs and teach them the necessary skills for participating in activities in their social environments. The basic CRA procedures include eight components: "functional analysis of substance use" that probes into the antecedents and consequences of the client's substance use; "sobriety sampling" that records the periods of alcohol- or drug-free achieved by the client; "CRA treatment plan" that consists of a Happiness Scale that includes different aspects of life for the client to choose to improve through receiving counselling; "behavioural skills training" in problem-solving, communication skills and alcohol/drug refusal skills; "job skills training" for getting and keeping a job; "social and recreational counselling" that helps the client to find new social and recreational activities that do not involve alcohol or drug use; "relapse prevention" that helps the client to prevent and cope with a relapse; and "relationship counselling" that helps the client to improve his/her interaction with his/her partner (Meyers et al. 2011). Among the above eight procedures, the Happiness Scale in the "CRA treatment plan" is a core element of the whole scheme, as it provides a basis for the design of a specific treatment for a client and serves as a yardstick for assessing the outcome of the treatment.

We have described some of the examples that quality of life or subjective well-being has recently been incorporated into treatment approaches overseas. They should inspire treatment workers and researchers in Hong Kong to recognize the increasingly important role of subjective well-being in drug treatment and rehabilitation. Apart from digging into the relationship between subjective well-being and drug use, its potential role as a treatment outcome should also be explored. Such a project would at least involve the search for an appropriate definition of subjective well-being, development of a valid scale for measuring subjective well-being, adoption of subjective well-being in treatment modules, formulation of criteria for the assessment of subjective well-being as an outcome of treatment, conducting of evaluative research on the results of treatments involving subjective well-being as an outcome, and mobilization of financial and manpower resources for the planning and implementation of this project. For this great step forward in drug treatment and rehabilitation services in Hong Kong, service providers, educationists, health professionals, policy makers, researchers, and scholars should join hands.

References

Bogart, L. M., Collins, R. L., Ellickson, P. L., & Klein, D. J. (2007). Are adolescent substance users less satisfied with life as young adults and if so, why? *Social Indicators Research, 81*, 149–169.

Brockmann, H., Delhey, J., Welzel, C., & Yuan, H. (2009). The China puzzle: Falling happiness in a rising economy. *Journal of Happiness Studies, 10*, 387–405.

Chen, Z., & Davey, G. (2008). Happiness and subjective wellbeing in mainland China. *Journal of Happiness Studies, 9*, 589–600.

Cheung, Y. W. (2009). *A brighter side: Protective and risk factors in the rehabilitation of chronic drug abusers in Hong Kong*. Hong Kong: The Chinese University Press.

Cummins, R. (2003). Normative life satisfaction: Measurement issues and a homeostatic model. *Social Indicators Research, 64*, 225–256.

Diener, E., & Diener, M. (1995). Cross-cultural correlates of life satisfaction and self-esteem. *Journal of Personality and Social Psychology, 68*(4), 653–663.

Diener, E., Emmons, R. A., Larsen, R. J., & Griffin, S. (1985). The life satisfaction scale. *Journal of Personality Assessment, 49*, 71–75.

Huebner, E. S. (2004). Research on assessment of life satisfaction of children and adolescents. *Social Indicators Research, 66*(1–2), 3–33.

Inoguchi, T., & Fujii, S. (2013). *The quality of life in Asia*. Dordrecht: Springer.

Ip, P. K., & Cheung, Y. W. (2014). Probing folk happiness in Taiwan. *Social Indicators Research, 117*, 689–703.

Lee, R. P. L., Cheung, T. S., & Cheung, Y. W. (1979). Material and non-material conditions and life satisfaction of urban residents in Hong Kong. In T. B. Lin, R. P. L. Lee, & U. E. Simons (Eds.), *Hong Kong: Economic, social and political studies in development* (pp. 83–94). White Plains: M.E. Sharpe.

Liao, P. S. (2009). Parallels between objective indicators and subjective perceptions of quality of life: A study of metropolitan and county areas in Taiwan. *Social Indicators Research, 91*, 99–114.

Maeyer, J. D., Vanderplasschen, W., & Broekaert, E. (2009). Exploratory study on drug users' perspectives on quality of life: More than health-related quality of life? *Social Indicators Research, 90*, 107–126.

Meyers, R. J., Villanueva, M., & Smith, J. E. (2005). The community reinforcement approach: History and new directions. *Journal of Cognitive Psychotherapy, 19*(3), 251–264.

Meyers, R. J., Roozen, H. G., & Smith, J. E. (2011). The community reinforcement approach: An update of the evidence. *Alcohol Research & Health, 33*(4), 380–388.

Proctor, C. L., Linley, P. A., & Maltby, J. (2009). Youth life satisfaction: A review of the literature. *Journal of Happiness Studies, 10*, 583–630.

Schalock, R. (1996). *Quality of life. Volume 1: Conceptualization and measurement*. Washington, DC: American Association on Mental Retardation.

Seligman, M. E. P. (2002). *Authentic happiness: Using the new positive psychology to realize your potential for lasting fulfillment*. New York: Free Press.

Shek, D. T. L. (1997). Family environment and adolescent psychological well-being, school adjustment, and problem behavior: A pioneer study in a Chinese context. *Journal of Genetic Psychology, 158*(1), 113–128.

Shek, D. T. L. (2002). Family environment and psychological well-being, school adjustment, and problem behavior in Chinese adolescents with and without economic disadvantage. *Journal of Genetic Psychology, 163*(4), 497–502.

Shek, D. T. L. (2003). Economic stress, psychological well-being and problem behavior in Chinese adolescents with economic disadvantage. *Journal of Youth and Adolescence, 32*(4), 259–266.

Shek, D. T. L. (2010). Introduction: Quality of life of Chinese people in a changing world. *Social Indicators Research, 95*, 357–361.

Shek, D. T. L., & Hollister, R. M. (Eds.). (2017). *University social responsibility: A global survey of concepts and experiences*. Singapore: Springer Nature.

Shek, D. T. L., & Liu, T. T. (2014). Life satisfaction in junior secondary school students in Hong Kong: A 3-year longitudinal study. *Social Indicators Research, 117*, 777–794.

Shek, D. T. L., Chan, Y. K., & Lee, P. S. N. (Eds.). (2005). *Quality of life research in Chinese, Western and global contexts*. Dordrecht: Springer.

Shu, X., & Zhu, Y. (2009). The quality of life in China. *Social Indicators Research, 92*, 191–225.

Sing, M. (2009). The quality of life in Hong Kong. *Social Indicators Research, 92*, 191–225.

Smith, K. W., & Larson, M. J. (2003). Quality of life assessments by adult substance abusers receiving publicly funded treatment in Massachusetts. *American Journal of Drug Alcohol Abuse, 29*, 323–335.

Smyth, R., Nielsen, I., & Zhai, Q. (2010). Personal well-being in urban China. *Social Indicators Research, 95*, 213–251.

Sun, R. C. F., & Shek, D. T. L. (2010). Life satisfaction, positive youth development, and problem behavior among Chinese adolescents in Hong Kong. *Social Indicators Research, 95*, 455–474.

Sun, R. C. F., & Shek, D. T. L. (2012). Positive youth development, life satisfaction and problem behavior among Chinese adolescents in Hong Kong: A replication. *Social Indicators Research, 105*, 541–559.

Tiffany, S. T., Friedman, L., Greenfied, S. F., Hasin, D. S., & Jackson, R. (2011). Beyond drug use: A systematic consideration of other outcomes in evaluations of treatments for substance use disorders. *Addiction, 107*, 709–718.

Torrens, M. (2008). Quality of life as a means of assessing outcome in opioid dependence treatment. *Heroin Addiction Related Clinical Problems, 11*, 33–36.

Tsou, M. W., & Liu, J. T. (2001). Happiness and domain satisfaction in Taiwan. *Journal of Happiness Studies, 2*, 269–288.

Valois, R. F., Zullig, K. J., Huebner, E. S., & Drane, J. W. (2004). Life satisfaction and suicide among high school adolescents. *Social Indicators Research, 66*, 81–105.

Wan, P. S., Law, K. W. K., & Wong, T. K. Y. (2008). Subjective well-being, 1997–2006. In S. W. Leung, P. S. Wan, & S. L. Wong (Eds.), *Indicators of social development: Hong Kong 2006* (pp. 209–244). Hong Kong: Hong Kong Institute of Asia-Pacific Studies, The Chinese University of Hong Kong.

Wu, C. H. (2009). Enhancing quality of life by shifting importance perception among life domains. *Journal of Happiness Studies, 10*(1), 37–47.

Ye, M., Li, L., Li, Y., Shen, R., Wen, S., & Zhang, J. (2013). Life satisfaction of adolescents in Hunan, China: Reliability and validity of Chinese brief multidimensional students' life satisfaction scale (BMSLSS). *Social Indicators Research, 118*(2), 515–522.

Zullig, K. J., Valois, R. F., Huebner, E. S., Oeltmann, J. E., & Drane, J. W. (2001). Relationship between perceived life satisfaction and adolescents' substance abuse. *Journal of Adolescent Health, 29*, 279–288.

Chapter 6
Summary and Discussion

The Study

This book has reported the findings of a longitudinal study of psychoactive drug users conducted by the senior author from 2009 to 2012, a time when the use of psychoactive drugs by young people in Hong Kong had drastically risen since the late 1990s. By that time, there was an increase of clinical research on the harmful physical and mental consequences of ketamine, the most dominant psychoactive drug in the past two decades. But little was known about the social characteristics of ketamine users and the demographic and psychological factors associated with their use. The 3-year longitudinal study addressed these and other issues by recruiting a sample of psychoactive drug users from 36 youth outreach as well as treatment and rehabilitation agencies. It was also a pioneer study of psychoactive drug use in Chinese settings that adopted a longitudinal design that allows the causality among variables to be assessed (Cheung 2012). A total of six interviews, spaced out at 6-month intervals, were conducted. The sample size of the baseline survey at T1 was 754, decreasing to 600 at T2, 434 at T3, 376 at T4, 347 at T5, and 288 at T6. The attrition rates towards the last rounds of interviews tended to be high, mainly due to case closure of clients (subjects) or premature departure of clients from the treatment and rehabilitation programmes. The sample at T1 mainly consisted of young people (mean age was 20.6), men (65.8%), and unmarried people (88.8%), with lower secondary school education and living in public housing, quite consistent with the social image of young psychoactive drug users in Hong Kong.

The major dependent variable was "drug use in the last 30 days" (yes or no), which showed the continuation or discontinuation of drug use at a time point. A number of commonly used socio-demographic and psychosocial variables were tested for their possible effects on the dependent variable at all six time points. Data of the second to the sixth time points were stacked into an individual time point structure. Random-effects probit regression was used to estimate the relative contributions of the dependent variables to the binary dependent variable of drug use in

Y.W. Cheung, N.W.-t. Cheung, *Psychoactive Drug Abuse in Hong Kong*,
Quality of Life in Asia 11, DOI 10.1007/978-981-10-6154-7_6

the last 30 days. The criterion for selection of independent variables into a regression was that the bivariate relationship between the independent variable and the dependent variable must be significant at four or more time points out of the total six time points. For the present analysis, subjects who were undergoing treatment in a programme would be excluded because no drug use was allowed in treatment settings and their drug-free condition might thus be artificial.

Socio-demographic and Psychosocial Correlates of Continuation of Drug Use

Our analysis first examined and compared how socio-demographic variables and psychosocial variables influenced the continuation/discontinuation of drug use. Socio-demographic variables used were as follows:

- Gender
- Age
- Whether or not a student
- Marital status
- Having a religion or not
- Housing type

Psychosocial variables included the following:

- Permissiveness to drug use
- Permissiveness to regular drug use
- Permissiveness to occasional drug use
- Educational strain
- Experience of discrimination
- Sense of uncertainty about future
- Think that doing extreme things shows the vitality of young people
- Wish to have own family, job, and normal life in future
- Think that parents don't know how to teach children
- Think that school doesn't know how to teach students
- Life satisfaction
- Self-esteem
- Depression
- Stricken by stressful events
- Subjective weathering

The "number of years of drug use", as an indication of drug use history, was also included, for the purpose of examining if drug use history affected the continuation or discontinuation of drug use.

Results of bivariate associations showed that none of the socio-demographic variables was significantly related to drug use in the last 30 days at four or more time points. Thus, socio-demographic variables were regarded as poor predictors of the continuation or discontinuation of drug use. In a way, that was not a surprising finding. As the "normalization of recreational drug use" perspective (Parker et al. 1998; Aldridge et al. 2011; Cheung and Cheung 2006) has pointed out, recreational or occasional drug use has become much more widely accepted and practised among young people than before, regardless of socio-demographic backgrounds. The lack of effects of socio-demographic variables is not limited to the initiation of drug use but also subsequent continuation of drug use.

Several focus group sessions had been conducted in the study. One of the interesting findings from our focus group discussions pertained to the non-significance of socio-demographic factors in predicting drug use. When a group of Form 1 to Form 3 male students were asked whether girls in school also snorted ketamine, one of them immediately replied that:

> Lots of girls played with ketamine nowadays! May be even more so than boys. The world has changed.

In another group, a participant said that:

> Band One schools also have students snorting K. They don't necessarily do it inside their schools, and so they are not caught by teachers.

Participants of a focus group comprising older (aged between 25 and 30) users who were working youths pointed out that ketamine use also cut across a wide spectrum of occupations, including taxi drivers, truck drivers (especially trucks that cross the boundary between Hong Kong and Shenzhen everyday), garage workers, moving service workers, construction site workers, restaurant kitchen workers, salespersons, and even real estate agents. The major reason for snorting K was to boost up their energy levels before starting to work. This required the use of an accurate dosage that was enough to "wake them up" but would not get them "exploded" (becoming difficult to control oneself due to overuse).

Psychosocial variables were much better predictors of continuation/discontinuation of drug use. Results of random-effects probit regression analysis showed that permissiveness to regular drug use, permissiveness to occasional drug use, life satisfaction, and depression were significantly related to drug use in the last 30 days. As the study collected panel data, our regression models also included variables at the previous time point. Drug use in the last 30 days at the previous time point, as well as self-esteem at the previous time point, significantly affected drug use in the last 30 days at the concurrent time point.

Since the above-mentioned psychosocial variables would have cross-sectional and/or longitudinal influence on drug use in the last 30 days, we further examined how they affected each other, because through affecting each other, they would also have indirect effects on continuation/discontinuation of drug use. Thus, regression models were tested for the two permissiveness to drug use variables, life satisfaction, self-esteem, and depression, respectively, as outcome variables and with other psychosocial variables as independent variables.

In addition, although socio-demographic variables were generally not significantly related to continuation/discontinuation of drug use, we had also examined whether there were any gender differences in how the psychosocial variables have affected drug use in the last 30 days and how the psychosocial variables have affected each other. The regressions performed for the whole sample were repeated for both the male and female subsamples, respectively.

In the following, we highlight and discuss each of the significant psychosocial variables, with illustrations from data obtained from the five focus group sessions conducted for the study.

Permissiveness to Drug Use

In this study, we have differentiated permissiveness to drug use into regular drug use and occasional drug use, in order to gauge the difference in effects on continuous drug use between these two prodrug attitudes. Both attitudes were strong predictors of continuation of drug use, although permissiveness towards occasional drug use cast a greater influence on the continuation of drug use than permissiveness to regular drug use, due to the popularity of the recreational form of drug use. In our sample of psychoactive drug users, as many as 79.5% of the subjects disagreed that drug use was an inappropriate behaviour, and 71.1% said that using drugs on recreational occasions was acceptable (T1 data). Why did psychoactive drug users hold a permissive attitude towards drug use?

In Chap. 1, we have already discussed the drug subculture of neutralization of recreational drug use among young psychoactive drug users in Hong Kong, which involved a negative evaluation of heroin and defining drug use as a bad habit rather than a drug problem. Let us revisit this phenomenon here with illustrations from focus group sessions. When it comes to adolescents' learning and practice of risk behaviour, the influence of peers is always on the centre stage. The first drug use never occurs in a vacuum; it tends to happen on a social occasion where friends are using the drug and the individual is persuaded to join in and try. To be sure, the experience of the first use of a drug is seldom a pleasant one, whether the drug is ketamine, ice, marijuana, or other psychoactive drugs. Many kinds of physical rejections (vomiting, nausea, etc.) could happen. However, the fun of doing drugs is very much a socially learned experience (Becker 1963). Once this "rite of passage" is fulfilled, drug use becomes a routine activity in gatherings with friends. As a Form 3 male student remarked in a focus group session:

> There is no fixed time in a day for snorting K (ketamine). Whenever some friends gather, we'll do it together…It is part of our daily activities. Whenever we are bored, we'll do drugs.

For drug-using youngsters, they come across lots of frustrations and unpleasant experiences every day. Friends' support becomes a very important basis for them to stick together. Psychoactive drug use very often serves as a source of peer support. As a young female described:

> Try the drug (ketamine) if you're feeling sad. You'll be okay after taking it. Aren't we friends?

Adolescence is a stage of life at which peers' influence is a lot greater than that of the family and school. This is especially true for the involvement in deviant behaviour (Cheung 1997; Johnson 1979; Thio 2010). Drug-using adolescents naturally flock together and rely heavily on each other for warm feelings and a sense of security, as a coping mechanism in the harsh reality they live in. The dependence on friends quickly leads to the dependence on drugs. The use of drugs is part of daily social life. It has become a habit. It has become something you always do, just like, as a focus group participant described, "eating snacks—chips, candies, etc.". Another participant remarked that he was so used to taking ketamine that the first thing he did when he woke up every day was not to brush his teeth or wash his face but to snort K. A female focus group participant said that she would use it even when she was taking a shower.

According to most participants of our focus group sessions, the dependence was more psychological than physical. They maintained that psychoactive drug use would not result in the kind of addiction problems that accompany heroin use. Heroin abuse would necessarily entail the craving for heroin every day. To young drug users, heroin was a "real drug", so terrifying that they would not try. A female focus group member described heroin use as a "road of no return". The Form 3 student user in another focus group firmly claimed that it was okay to play with different psychoactive drugs, but heroin was a definite "no", because the scenario of heroin injection was too frightening.

However, the awareness of the serious consequences of heroin addiction was, unfortunately, a double-edged sword. The positive side of it was that there seemed to be a common understanding and practice among young drug users that heroin should not be touched. The negative side was that it lowered their awareness of the danger of psychoactive drugs. Many of them thought that psychoactive drugs were not very addictive, so that they could enter and exit drug use whenever they wished. Thus, they thought that as long as they did not do heroin, they would be safe. Indeed, many of our focus group participants have pointed out that they have not suffered many withdrawal symptoms from stopping ketamine use. At most, minor discomforts such as a runny nose might occur, but they were a lot milder than the pain due to the craving for heroin. It was easier to stop psychoactive drug use than to stop heroin use. This, true as it may be, was, however, a trap. Addiction is not only a matter of physical dependence. Psychological dependence may even be more difficult to overcome. As youngsters develop the habit of psychoactive drug use, psychological dependence quickly accumulates, making drug use more and more ingrained into their daily lives. Interestingly, ketamine users in the focus groups introduced me to a term they used to describe their psychological dependence on the drug—"nostril dependence". That was a very vivid description! One of them said that if on a certain day she couldn't satisfy the desire of her nose to snort ketamine, she would become very uptight and impatient the whole day.

The "habit" of psychoactive drug use, a consequence of psychological dependence, was facilitated by the easy availability of the drug and the convenience in its consumption. As a 24-year-old male focus group participant described:

> You call him (supplier), and he will drive to deliver whatever quantity you want. Very easy.

Snorting ketamine was also a very convenient mode of administration of the drug. As a participant of a female focus group session remarked:

> It was easy to snort K inside the classroom by laying your head on the desk. You can also do it inside the school toilet. You just wash your nose with water afterwards.

Another participant said:

> If you are skillful enough, you can snort K while walking on the street or at the toilet of your workplace.

As pointed out in Chap. 1, the misconception that psychoactive drugs are much less addictive than heroin, and thus much less dangerous, provided the justification for young drug users not to be alerted to the harms of acquiring the habit of psychoactive drug use. To be sure, many of them admitted that taking ketamine or other psychoactive drugs was a *bad habit*. However, bad habits were very common, especially among energetic and reckless adolescents. Many young people had lots of bad habits, such as excessively playing computer games, gambling, drinking, smoking, gang fighting, absence from school, speaking foul languages, premarital sex, theft, vandalism, etc. Snorting ketamine was no more than one of the common bad habits. This reduction of drug abuse to bad habit, or what we have called "bad habitization" (Cheung and Zhong 2014), could result in a low degree of awareness of the danger of psychoactive drug abuse, a stubbornly high level of permissiveness to drug use, and the denial of having a "drug problem", not to mention the lack of motivation to seek treatment.

In the whole sample, permissiveness to occasional drug use was found to be a stronger predictor for continuation/discontinuation of drug use than was permissiveness to regular use. The same finding was present in both the male and female subsamples, but among females, the effect of permissiveness to occasional drug use was even greater than that of males. Furthermore, unlike males, females' permissiveness to regular drug use was not significantly related to drug use. These findings showed that there were gender differences in how prodrug attitudes affected drug use. If anything, more and more females were moving away from the traditional female drug user image of misery and victimization to catching up with males in pleasure seeking through recreational drug use. Such gender differences should be considered in intervention efforts that seek to change the permissive attitudes towards drug use among drug users.

Important as they might be, the permissive attitudes at the previous time point did not exert influence on drug use at the concurrent time point for both male and female groups. If the effects of the attitudes did not necessarily persist across the time points, then there was a greater chance of changing the attitudes from one time point to the next. However, the other side of the same coin is that improved attitudes would not necessarily last, so that efforts must be kept up in order to sustain positive changes of attitudes achieved previously.

Lastly, gender differences also existed in how the two attitudes were affected by other psychosocial variables. For males, the adventurous view of doing extreme things shows the vitality of young people, the conforming view of wishing to have own family, job, and normal life in future, the negative view of school, and life satisfaction had been significantly related to permissiveness to regular and/or permissiveness to occasional drug use. But for females, none of these psychosocial variables were good predictors of their permissive attitudes, except that the adventurous view of doing extreme things showing vitality of young people was significantly related to permissiveness to occasional drug use. More research is needed to find out factors that influence females' prodrug attitudes.

This study has employed some of the major ideas in the "normalization of recreational drug use" thesis (Parker et al. 1998) in organizing its conceptual framework and interpreting some of its findings. The two attitudinal variables of permissiveness to occasional and regular drug use are an important component of the normalization thesis, as the increasing acceptance of recreational drug use by young people is a necessary condition for normalization. The finding in this study that permissiveness to occasional drug use has even a greater influence on continuous drug use than permissiveness to regular drug use further illustrates the strong appeal of occasional drug use as young people make reasoned choices in their drug use as a normal part of leisure. The lack of significant relationships between socio-demographic variables and continuation/discontinuation of drug use echoes the point made by the normalization thesis that differences in the socio-demographic background are no longer good predictors of drug use.

However, this study also addressed a major weakness of the normalization thesis, which is its inability to make predictions about future patterns of drug use beyond normalization[1] (Asbridge et al. 2016; Williams 2016). If adolescent drug users make drug-wise choices of moderate use in recreational settings during their adolescence, what would be their pattern of use after they transition to young adulthood? Will they stop use, maintain recreational use, or progress to problematic use as they

[1] Other weaknesses of the normalization thesis include (i) failure to consider the influence of social structural factors, such as socioeconomic and cultural conditions, social networks, and law enforcement, on the extent and patterns of normalization among different youth groups and (ii) tendency to exaggerate the extent of social and cultural accommodation of recreational drug use (Fitzgerald et al. 2013; Williams 2016). As normalization varies in terms of extent and with the types of drugs used by different youth groups, some scholars preferred the term "differentiated normalization" (Shildrick 2002; Shiner and Newburn 1997) to the simplistic and uniform view of normalization in youth drug use. MacDonald and Marsh's (2002) study of youth in a socially exclude neighbourhood in Northeast England showed that abstinence, recreational use, and problematic use coexisted. In Hong Kong, Cheung and Cheung's (2006) finding that normalization was limited to marginal youths rather than a widespread phenomenon in the whole youth population is another example of differentiated normalization.

become young adults? These three possible outcomes represent three "trajectories" of adolescent drug use (Maggs et al. 2013; Hser et al. 2007). The first two trajectories (i.e. from recreational drug use in adolescence to stopping use in adulthood and from recreational drug use in adolescence to continuation of recreational use when entering young adulthood) can be mapped out by conducting a community survey of young adults who had used drugs in their adolescence. Their current reported patterns of drug use can be compared with their reported use during adolescence. A disadvantage of this method is that young drug-using adults who are in treatment programmes or correctional facilities could not be included in the community survey. As these young adults can be found in treatment and correctional agencies, the third trajectory (from recreational drug use in adolescence to problematic use in young adulthood) can be discerned by studying the changes in the patterns of drug use since adolescence among young adult clients of these agencies. The three trajectories warrant a new round of international research to shed light on new developments of the normalization thesis.

Life Satisfaction and Depression

The second most significant independent variable affecting psychoactive drug use was life satisfaction. Subjects who were more satisfied with their lives were less likely to have used psychoactive drugs in the last 30 days. Depression yielded a significant, but much weaker, relationship with drug use. Subjects with a higher degree of depression were more likely to continue drug use. Life satisfaction and depression were used to illustrate the broader concept of subjective well-being. The increasingly important role played by subjective well-being in treatment and rehabilitation programmes has been discussed in Chap. 5.

Self-Esteem

Self-esteem could not be said to be a strong predictor for continuation/discontinuation of psychoactive drug use, as it did not yield any significant relationship with drug use in the last 30 days at the concurrent time point, for the whole sample as well as the two gender groups. Interestingly enough, the effect of self-esteem was causal, as self-esteem at the previous time point strongly affected drug use in the last 30 days at the current time point for the male group but not the female group. This gender difference, possibly due to gender role socialization in which males are more likely than females to be socialized with instrumental problem-solving capabilities as discussed in Chap. 4, should be noted in intervention strategies.

That self-esteem did not yield any significant relationship with drug use in the last 30 days suggested that it did not have any direct effect on drug use. However, this does not mean that indirect effects are necessarily absent. Self-esteem could affect other psychosocial factors which were significantly related to drug use, thereby indirectly affecting drug use. As mentioned earlier, self-esteem was significantly and strongly related to life satisfaction, which was a strong predictor of drug use in the last 30 days in both males and females. An improvement in self-esteem could raise the level of life satisfaction, thereby indirectly reducing the tendency of drug use. As self-esteem also affected depression, which strongly affected life satisfaction, and which strongly affected drug use, it can be said that self-esteem indirectly affected drug use.

Self-esteem was a very stable variable. Self-esteem at the previous time point significantly and strongly effected self-esteem at the concurrent time point. This was true for both gender groups. Change of self-esteem might involve greater efforts to achieve, but when change was achieved, it would be able to sustain.

The relationship between self-esteem and substance use or risk behaviour has not been a conclusive finding in the literature. This study provided a mild support to studies that did not find a significant association between low self-esteem and substance use (e.g. Jones and Heaven 1998; Moore et al. 1996) but suggested that its indirect effects on drug use or other deviant behaviour should be further examined.

Drug Use at Previous Time Point

In our regressions of psychosocial variables on drug use in the last 30 days for the whole sample as well as the two gender groups, drug use at the previous time point was a very strong and significant variable. The finding of the powerful influence of drug use at one time point on drug use at the next time point was only to be expected. The use of drugs at one time point indicated the strong presence of physical and psychological dependence at that time point, and so, unless such dependence was effectively removed by treatment, drug use would continue at the next time point. This finding was not limited to psychoactive drug use in young people. In the above-mentioned longitudinal study of chronic adult drug abusers conducted by the senior author 10 years before the present study, drug use in one 12-month interval also directly affected drug use in the next 12-month interval (Cheung 2009).

Short-Term Effects of Psychosocial Variables

Through our longitudinal survey data, we have observed that none of the psychosocial variables had exerted any direct effects on drug use at the next time point, with the exception of self-esteem at the previous time point for the male group. In other words, the influence of the psychosocial variables was mostly short term, limited to affecting drug use within the same time point. Very seldom were they able to affect drug use at subsequent time points.

The short-term effect of independent variables on drug use had both an advantage and a disadvantage. The advantage was that the adverse effects of the psychosocial variables (high level of permissiveness to regular or occasional drug use, lack of life satisfaction, low self-esteem, and high level of depression) on drug use would not spill over to the next time point. Thus, at the next time point, there would be room for intervention or secondary/tertiary prevention work to improve the relevant psychosocial variables in order to reduce the likelihood of drug use. In other words, there was always hope for reducing the tendency to use drugs at the next time point. The other side of the same coin was the disadvantage that even if drug use was discontinued at one time point through improving the psychosocial variables, the good result would not automatically carry over to the next time point. Every time point was a new battlefield. Good intervention work must be kept up in order that positive results could sustain.

Epilogue

We have summarized and discussed the major findings of the "Longitudinal Survey of Psychoactive Drug Abusers in Hong Kong" (LSPDA) conducted from 2009 to 2012, as well as their service implications for young psychoactive drug users. Before we end, it is worthwhile to refer again to the "Longitudinal Study of Chronic Drug Abusers in Hong Kong" (LSCDA) (Cheung 2009), which we have mentioned in the last chapter. A comparison of these two longitudinal studies can reflect the changes in Hong Kong's drug scene in the last two decades.

The first longitudinal study of drug abusers in Hong Kong, LSCDA was conducted by the senior author, with the assistance of the second author, almost 10 years before LSPDA (2000–2003) for the former and 2009–2012 for the latter). As described earlier, subjects for LSCDA were selected from outreach agencies and drug treatment and rehabilitation programmes according to criteria of having a minimum of 5 years of addiction history and having had at least two relapses in the past. Three waves of interviews were conducted, spaced out at 12-month intervals. The size of the baseline sample obtained at the first wave of interviews was 547 subjects, and those for the samples of the second and third waves of interviews were 401 and 319, respectively. The dependent variable showing drug use/drug-free status was operationalized as "percentage of drug-free weeks", which was the percentage of weeks that the subject was drug-free among the total number of weeks that he/she was not in a residential programme in the interval concerned. A variety of psychosocial variables (self-efficacy, association with drug-using friends, life satisfaction, job attitude, etc.) were used to find out their strengths in predicting percentage of drug-free weeks.

The mean age of the baseline sample of LSCDA was 36.3, whereas that of LSPDA was 20.6. Among LSCDA subjects, 66% took heroin/opium as the first drug, but 93% of subjects in LSPDA had used ketamine or other psychoactive drugs as their first drugs. These two samples practically represented two generations of drugs and drug abusers. LSCDA subjects who belonged to the older age groups in the sample were probably the last batch of the older generation drug addicts who mainly abused heroin, in contrast to the majority of LSPDA subjects who represented the new generation of drug users who primarily rejected heroin and used ketamine or other psychoactive drugs.

The difference between these two generations of drug users went beyond the change of the drug of choice from heroin to ketamine. We have argued in Chap. 1 that the pattern of drug use has been shaped by the social change in Hong Kong that has occurred in the past several decades. The beginning of popularity of recreational psychoactive drug use among young people in the 1990s coincided with a time when Hong Kong had undergone the restructuring of economy from manufacturing to a globalized financial economy, the weakening of traditional cultural values and informal social control of adolescents by parents and teachers, and the rise of individualism and consumerism. Faced with high competition and uncertainty of the future, more and more young people were involved in recreational drug use as a way to respond to tough reality, and their attitude towards drug use became more and more permissive. The normalization of recreational drug use in Hong Kong has the additional unique feature of young people neutralizing the use of ketamine and other psychoactive drugs by rejecting heroin. The change of the drug of choice represented a change of drug subculture, which, in turn, was shaped by the change of social and cultural conditions in society.

How will young people's drug subculture change in future? Will there be a new wave of drug use involving a new category of drugs, comparable to the drastic change from heroin to ketamine in the late 1990s? In order to know the answers, more in-depth research is needed to find out how the youth drug subculture is changing in Hong Kong. At the individual drug user's level, what are the process and techniques of neutralization (Sykes and Matza 1957; Matza 1964) employed by young drug users to prefer certain drugs to others and to manage the stigmatized identity associated with illicit psychoactive drug use in mainstream society (Hathaway et al. 2011; Sznitman 2008; Pennay and Moore 2010)? How do young users negotiate risks associated with recreational and heavier consumption of the psychoactive drugs of their choice (Hunt et al. 2007; Singer and Schensul 2011). At the society level, Hong Kong is experiencing unprecedentedly huge and divisive conflicts in its sociopolitical developments. Many members of the younger generation are disgruntled with limited upward mobility as well as upholding universal values of democracy and justice. The tide is rising for these young people to be attracted to radical ideology and engage in street demonstrations and other means of protests, in which the use of violence has now become a norm. How will the political turbulences in the society and rising youth militancy impact on the general youth population? Will these social and political unrests affect the drug subculture in youth, and if they will, in what way?

As social conditions change, young people's drug subculture may also change. Behind the changes, however, there seems to be a common feature between them. Each drug subculture may be viewed as a means whereby young people adapt to stress and hardship in life in a particular period. The idea of drug use being an adaptation to harsh life is by no means new, but the "dislocation theory" recently proposed by the psychologist, Bruce Alexander, is worth noting. The theory stipulates that an individual's drug addiction is an adaptation to his/her experience of being dislocated at psychological and social levels living in a distorted world under the global dominance of the free market economy (Alexander 2008). Although Alexander did not address Parker's normalization perspective in his theory, the concepts of dislocation and adaptation fit very well with young people's increasing acceptance and involvement in drug use as a response to living in a risk society full of uncertainties and competition. Recreational use of psychoactive drugs among young people in Hong Kong could be seen as a way to adapt to the social change that has occurred in Hong Kong in the past two or three decades.

If drug use is an adaptation to a psychosocially distorted world, or to a risk society, then those people who feel the need to find an adaptation would likely be having a low level of life satisfaction. It was hardly surprising, therefore, that in both the older sample of LSCDA and the younger sample of LSPDA, life satisfaction was a significant and strong predictor of continuous drug use. Perhaps life satisfaction may be seen as a barometer for the tendency of drug users to continue to engage in drug use as a means of adaptation. This study (LSPDA) has examined how a drug user's life satisfaction might affect his/her continuation or discontinuation of drug use. In the previous chapter, we have discussed the prospect for subjective well-being to be incorporated as a treatment outcome in treatment and rehabilitation programmes. The role of subjective well-being in the change of youth drug subculture, in the context of normalization of recreational drug use or societal dislocation, is another high-priority agenda item in the future research of young people's drug use in Hong Kong.

Limitations of the Study

Several limitations of the study pertaining to the design and conduct of the study (Cheung 2012) were as follows:

1. The criterion for selecting subjects of agencies was having ever abused any psychoactive drugs. There was no differentiation of new users, occasional users, regular users, or heavy and problematic users in the subjects recruited. It was impossible to identify and determine the size of so diverse and heterogeneous a target population. Obtained in this way, the sample was necessarily a non-probability one. We had tried to improve the representativeness of the sample by recruiting as many subjects as possible and from as many as agencies as possible.
2. The study relied on social workers of the participating agencies to serve as interviewers of subjects recruited from their respective agencies. While there were pros and cons in this arrangement, it was difficult to estimate how much bias

might have occurred due to social desirability effect, i.e. the tendency for subjects to under-report their drug use in front of their social workers.

3. The questionnaire of the survey was meant to be short, for the practical reasons of easy administration of the interviews by agency staff and suiting the short concentration span of drug using subjects in interviews. The analysis would have been richer if some other useful psychosocial variables (e.g. self-efficacy, association with drug using friends) had been included in the questionnaire.
4. The overall drop-out rate was quite high, especially at T3, which was 12 months after the first wave of interviews had been conducted. High drop-out rates were not unexpected, as departures from the agencies, whether due to completion of service or premature quitting of service, happened all the time. Moreover, in this analysis, subjects who were in a residential agency at the time of interview would not be included in the analysis, thereby further reducing the number of subjects included in the analysis.

The following limitations lied in the measurement of variables and statistical analysis:

1. The major conceptual thread of the study was normalization of recreational drug use. In the questionnaire, occasional drug use was asked, but the questions did not really assess recreational drug use. Occasional use only described the frequency of use but said nothing about the purpose of use. It was only an assumption that occasional drug use would be associated with recreational drug use rather than heavy drug use.
2. The major dependent variable of drug use in the last 30 days was measured with a yes-no dichotomy. More in-depth analysis of drug use could have been made if information on the frequency of use and quantity of drugs was also collected.
3. Independent variables selected for inclusion into probit regressions were each required to have a significant bivariate relationship with the dependent variable concerned for at least four out of the six time points. While this practice seemed to have face validity, there was a certain degree of arbitrariness in it, and there were no statistical justifications to back it up.

References

Aldridge, J., Measham, F., & Willams, L. (2011). *Illegal leisure revisited: Changing patterns of alcohol and drug use in adolescents and young adults*. New York: Routledge.

Asbridge, M., Valleriani, J., Kwok, J., & Erickson, P. G. (2016). Normalization and denormalization in different legal contexts: Comparing cannabis and tobacco. *Drugs: Education, Prevention and Policy, 23*(3), 212–223.

Alexander, B. (2008). *The globalization of addiction: A study in poverty of the spirit*. Oxford: Oxford University Press.

Becker, H. (1963). *Outsiders: Studies in the sociology of deviance*. New York: Free Press.

Cheung, N. W. T., & Cheung, Y. W. (2006). Is Hong Kong experiencing normalization of adolescent drug use? Some reflections on the normalization thesis. *Substance Use & Misuse, 41*(14), 1967–1990.

Cheung, Y. W. (1997). Family, school, peer and media predictors of adolescent deviant behavior in Hong Kong. *Journal of Youth and Adolescence, 26*(5), 569–596.

Cheung, Y. W. (2009). *A brighter side: Protective and risk factors in the rehabilitation of chronic drug abusers in Hong Kong*. Hong Kong: The Chinese University Press.

Cheung, Y. W. (2012). *A longitudinal survey of psychoactive drug abusers in Hong Kong*. Report submitted to Beat Drugs Fund, Narcotics Division, Security Bureau, Government of the Hong Kong SAR. In website of Narcotics Division: http://www.nd.gov.hk/pdf/Longitudinal%20Survey%20of%20Psychoactive%20Drug%20Abusers%20in%20Hong%20Kong%20-%20report.pdf. Access date: April 9, 2017.

Cheung, Y. W., & Zhong, S. H. (2014). Official reactions to crime and drug problems in Hong Kong. In C. Liqun, I. Sun, & B. Hebenton (Eds.), *The Routledge Handbook of Chinese Criminology* (pp. 295–308). Oxon: Routledge.

Fitzgerald, R., Mazerolle, L., & Mazerolle, P. (2013). Drug normalization and Australian youth: Group differences in the social accommodation of drug use. *Journal of Youth Studies, 16*, 901–915.

Hathaway, A., Comeau, N., & Erickson, P. (2011). Cannabis normalization and stigma: Contemporary practices of moral regulation. *Criminology and Criminal Justice, 11*, 451–469.

Hser, Y. I., Longshore, D., & Anglin, M. D. (2007). The life course perspective on drug use: A conceptual framework for understanding drug use trajectories. *Evaluation Review, 31*(6), 515–547.

Hunt, G., Moloney, M., & Evans, K. (2007). Drug use and meanings of risk and pleasure. *Journal of Youth Studies, 10*(1), 73–96.

Johnson, R. E. (1979). *Juvenile delinquency and its origins: An integrated theoretical approach*. Cambridge: Cambridge University Press.

Jones, S. P., & Heaven, P. C. L. (1998). Psychosocial correlates of adolescent drug-taking behaviour. *Journal of Adolescence, 21*(2), 127–134.

MacDonald, R., & Marsh, J. (2002). Crossing the Rubicon: Youth transitions, poverty, drugs and social exclusion. *International Journal of Drug Policy, 13*, 27–38.

Maggs, J. L., Wray-Lake, L., & Schulenberg, J. E. (2013). Developmental risk taking and the natural history of alcohol and drug use among youth. In P. M. Miller (Ed.), *Principles of addiction: Comprehensive addictive behaviors and disorders* (pp. 535–544). New York: Elsevier.

Matza, D. (1964). *Delinquency and drift*. New York: Wiley.

Moore, S., Laflin, M. T., & Weis, D. L. (1996). The role of cultural norms in the self-esteem and drug use relationship. *Adolescence, 31*, 523–542.

Parker, H., Aldridge, J., & Measham, F. (1998). *Illegal leisure: The normalization of adolescent recreational drug use*. London: Routledge.

Pennay, A. E., & Moore, D. (2010). Exploring the micro-politics of normalization: Narratives of pleasure, self-control and desire in a sample of young Australian 'party drug' users. *Addiction Research and Theory, 18*, 557–571.

Shildrick, T. (2002). Young people, illicit drug use and the question of normalization. *Journal of Youth Studies, 5*, 35–48.

Shiner, M., & Newburn, T. (1997). Definitely, maybe not? The normalization of recreational drug use amongst young people. *Sociology, 31*, 511–529.

Singer, E. O., & Schensul, J. J. (2011). Negotiating ecstasy risk, reward, and control: A qualitative analysis of drug management patterns among ecstasy-using urban young adults. *Substance Use & Misuse, 46*, 1675–1689.

Sykes, G., & Matza, D. (1957). Techniques of neutralization. *American Sociological Review, 22*, 664–670.

Sznitman, S. R. (2008). Drug normalization and the case of Sweden. *Contemporary Drug Problems, 35*, 447–580.

Thio, A. (2010). *Deviant behavior* (10th ed.). Boston: Allyn & Bacon.

Williams, L. (2016). Muddy waters?: Reassessing the dimensions of the normalization thesis in twenty-first century Britain. *Drugs: Education, Prevention and Policy, 23*(3), 190–201.

Appendices

Appendix One: A Closer Look at the Sample (Adopted from Cheung, Y.W. (2012). *A longitudinal survey of psychoactive drug abusers in Hong Kong*. Report submitted to Beat Drugs Fund, Narcotics Division, Security Bureau, Government of the Hong Kong SAR. pp. 114–122)

In Table 2.1, we have reported the size of the baseline sample at T1 and its changes from T2 to T6. Here, we take a look at the drop-out situation from T2 to T6 and discuss how it might have contributed to the biases of the sample. A "drop-out case" is broadly defined as a subject who was in the sample of a time point but was not in the sample at the next time point. The major reason for a subject to become a drop-out case at a time point is his/her departure from the agency (outreach/counselling or residential T&R) where he/she was a client at the previous time point. The subject might have left the agency prematurely, unwilling to finish the service period although still not drug-free; or he/she might have become drug-free upon completion of the service period.

Before we examine the drop-out situation at various time points, it must be pointed out that measures had been taken by all participating agencies to minimize the number of drop-out cases. Firstly, an effective system of managing interview matters for the longitudinal survey was designed and implemented by participating agencies, so as to gauge the maximum participation of subjects in each round of the interviews. Secondly, the adoption of the "suitable interview period" ("3 weeks before" and "3 weeks after" the designated interview date) also gave flexibility for interviews to be conducted in favour of the subjects' availability. Thirdly, the agency staff would try to maintain contact with subjects who had left the agency. They always had their ways of tracking down prematurely and maturely departed cases and motivating them to continue to participate in subsequent interviews. Fourthly, for those who had entered a CSD facility, efforts were made to interview them in the facility. Fifthly, at the end of the T3 interview, each subject was given a ball pen as

Y.W. Cheung, N.W.-t. Cheung, *Psychoactive Drug Abuse in Hong Kong*, Quality of Life in Asia 11, DOI 10.1007/978-981-10-6154-7 a small gift and a card reminding them the dates of the next and last three interviews. Lastly, the agencies agreed to recruit as many clients as possible for the baseline T1 sample, in order that, despite attrition, the sample size at the last time point would be big enough for statistical analysis. Without the help and efforts of the agencies, the attrition rates at the time points would have been much higher.

Next, we compare the subjects in the sample (retained subjects) and drop-out cases for each of the time points from T2 to T6.

Drop-Out Group at T2

For T2, we compare the socio-demographic characteristics and psychosocial conditions (only those most significantly related to drug use) at T1 of the retained subjects group (T2 sample) and the drop-out group. Results are reported in Table 1.

At T2, the number of retained subjects was 600, and the number of drop-outs was 154. The percentage of retention was 600/(600 + 154) = 79.6 %, and the percentage of attrition was 154/754 = 20.4 %.

The two groups were significantly different in several of the characteristics compared. In the drop-out group, there were higher percentages of male, subjects aged 21 or older, married subjects, and non-students than in the retained subjects group. Interestingly, the drop-out group had a much higher percentage (55.2 %) of being in residential agencies at T1, compared with 16.7 % in the retained subjects group. Moreover, a much higher percentage (63 %) of drop-outs did not use drugs at T1, whereas only 44.2 % of retained subjects were drug-free at T1.

The above findings suggest that many of the drop-outs were likely to be clients of residential T&R agencies who were able to become drug-free at T1 and had left these programmes by T2. These drop-out subjects were more likely than retained subjects to have a lower degree of permissiveness to drug use, although they had a longer history of drug abuse than retained subjects.

Drop-Out Group at T3

We next compare the retained subjects group and the drop-out group at T3, with respect to socio-demographic and psychosocial characteristics at T2 (Table 2).

At T3, the number of retained subjects was 434, and the number of drop-outs was 181. The percentage of retention was 434/(434 + 181) = 70.6 %, and the percentage of drop-outs was 181/615 = 29.4 %.

The two groups varied significantly in a number of socio-demographic and drug use characteristics. There were higher percentages of subjects aged 21 or older, with longer history of drug use, and with lower education in the drop-out group than in the retained subjects group. As to type of agency and drug use, the drop-out group had a higher percentage of residential programme clients at T2 than the retained subjects group.

Table 1 Comparison of retained subjects and drop-outs at T2

Socio-demographic and selected psychosocial variables *at T1*	T2 Retained subjects ($n = 600$)	T2 Drop-outs ($n = 154$)	N
Gender ($p <.05$)			754
M	63.8	73.4	496
F	36.2	26.6	258
Age ($p <.001$)			754
12–16	35.8	18.2	243
17–20	41.7	35.7	305
21 or over	22.5	46.1	206
No. of siblings (n.s.)			754
Marital status ($p <.001$)			752
Never married	91.5	78.4	668
Married	8.5	21.6	84
Education (n.s.)			753
Whether still a student ($p <.001$)			753
Yes, always attending school	25.5	13.6	174
Yes, but not always attending	8.0	3.2	53
No	66.4	83.1	526
Religion (n.s.)			752
Type of agency ($p <.001$)			754
Outreach/no agency	83.3	44.8	569
Residential	16.7	55.2	185
Drug use ($p <.001$)			753
No	44.2	63.0	362
Yes	55.8	37.0	391
No. of years of drug abuse ($p < .001$)			750
0–2	44.1	23.4	299
3–5	32.7	26.6	236
6 or more	23.3	50.0	215
Permissiveness to drug use ($p <.001$)			749
Low	37.0	55.2	305
Medium	52.3	41.6	375
High	10.8	3.2	69
Satisfaction with life (n.s.)			754
Self-esteem (n.s.)			753

Significance levels are based on χ^2 tests
n.s. not statistically significant

Table 2 Comparison of retained subjects and drop-outs at T3

Socio-demographic and selected psychosocial variables *at T2*	T3 Retained subjects (n = 434)	Drop-outs (n = 181)	N
Gender (n.s.)			615
Age ($p < .05$)			581
12–16	31.3	25.6	172
17–20	48.4	43.6	273
21 or over	20.3	30.8	136
No. of siblings (n.s.)			600
Marital status (n.s.)			600
Education ($p < .05$)			598
Primary – F3	59.0	68.0	369
F4–F5	36.2	30.9	207
Beyond F5	4.8	1.1	22
Whether still a student (n.s.)			600
Religion (n.s.)			569
Type of agency ($p < .001$)			600
Outreach/no agency	85.4	74.0	492
Residential	14.6	26.0	108
Drug use (n.s.)			599
No. of years of drug abuse ($p < .05$)			595
0–2	33.3	27.2	187
3–5	41.7	36.7	239
6 or more	25.1	36.1	169
Permissiveness to drug use (n.s.)			596
Satisfaction with life (n.s.)			600
Self-esteem (n.s.)			599

Significance levels are based on χ^2 tests
n.s. not statistically significant

Drop-Out Group at T4

Table 3 compares the socio-demographic and psychosocial characteristics of the two groups.

At T4, the number of retained subjects was 376, and the number of drop-outs was 95. The percentage of retention was 376/(376 + 95) = 79.8 %, and the drop-out rate was 95/471 = 20.2 %.

In terms of socio-demographic characteristics, the drop-out group at T4 differed from the drop-out groups at T2 and T3 in a few ways. Compared with the retained subjects group, it had a higher percentage of male, a smaller percentage of subjects having one or two siblings, and a higher percentage of subjects having a religion. Like at T2 and T3, the drop-out group at T4 also had a higher percentage of subjects aged 21 or older. It also had a higher percentage of subjects with a longer history of drug abuse. There is reason to believe that some of the dropped-out subjects at T4

Table 3 Comparison of retained subjects and drop-outs at T4

	T4		
Socio-demographic and selected psychosocial variables *at T3*	Retained subjects ($n = 376$)	Drop-outs ($n = 95$)	N
Gender ($p < .001$)			471
M	60.1	78.9	301
F	39.9	21.1	170
Age ($p < .05$)			434
12–16	25.4	14.7	100
17–20	51.1	42.1	220
21 or over	21.5	43.2	114
No. of siblings ($p < .01$)			471
0	9.8	22.1	58
1–2	72.3	57.9	327
3 or more	17.8	20.0	86
Marital status (n.s.)			434
Education (n.s.)			434
Whether still a student (n.s.)			434
Religion ($p < .001$)			434
No	74.6	53.7	304
Yes	25.4	46.3	130
Type of agency ($p < .001$)			434
Outreach/no agency	92.6	66.3	377
Residential	7.4	33.7	57
Drug use (n.s.)			434
No. of years of drug abuse ($p < .01$)			418
0–2	26.1	17.6	102
3–5	48.0	40.0	194
6 or more	25.8	42.4	122
Permissiveness to drug use ($p < .05$)			433
Low	46.4	60.0	214
Medium	46.4	37.9	193
High	7.1	2.1	26
Satisfaction with life (n.s.)			434
Self-esteem (n.s.)			434

Significance levels are based on χ^2 tests
n.s. not statistically significant

Table 4 Comparison of retained subjects and drop-outs at T5

Socio-demographic and selected psychosocial variables *at T4*	T5 Retained subjects ($n = 345$)	Drop-outs ($n = 67$)	N
Gender (n.s.)			412
Age (n.s.)			373
No. of siblings (n.s.)			412
Marital status (n.s.)			376
Education (n.s.)			376
Whether still a student (n.s.)			376
Religion (n.s.)			376
Type of agency (n.s.)			376
Drug use (n.s.)			376
No. of years of drug abuse ($p < .01$)			375
0–2	18.2	7.5	61
3–5	52.9	46.3	194
6 or more	28.9	46.3	120
Permissiveness to drug use (n.s.)			375
Satisfaction with life (n.s.)			376
Self-esteem ($p < .05$)			375
Low	23.0	22.7	86
Medium	23.6	39.4	99
High	53.4	37.9	190

Significance levels are based on χ^2 tests
n.s. not statistically significant

had left because they had finished residential programmes, as one-third of them were in residential T&R agencies at T3, and they had a higher percentage of subjects with a low level of permissiveness to drug use.

Drop-Out Group at T5

The drop-out group and retained subjects group at T5 are compared in Table 4.

At T5, the number of retained subjects was 345, and the number of drop-outs was 67. The percentage of retention was 345/(345 + 67) = 83.7 %, and the drop-out rate was 67/412 = 16.3 %.

The two groups were significantly different in only two of the characteristics. Like at all previous time points, the drop-out group at T5 had subjects with the longest history of drug abuse than the retained subjects group. Drop-outs were also more likely to have a lower level of self-esteem than retained subjects at T5.

Table 5 Comparison of retained subjects and drop-outs at T6

Socio-demographic and selected psychosocial variables *at T5*	T6 Retained subjects ($n = 286$)	Drop-outs ($n = 87$)	N
Gender ($p < .05$)			373
M	58.0	72.4	229
F	42.0	27.6	144
Age (n.s.)			341
No. of siblings (n.s.)			373
Marital status (n.s.)			344
Education (n.s.)			343
Whether still a student (n.s.)			344
Religion (n.s.)			344
Type of agency (n.s.)			345
Drug use (n.s.)			345
No. of years of drug abuse (n.s.)			343
Permissiveness to drug use (n.s.)			340
Satisfaction with life (n.s.)			345
Self-esteem (n.s)			345

Significance levels are based on $\chi 2$ tests
n.s. not statistically significant

Drop-Out Group at T6

Lastly, we examine the two groups at T6 (Table 5).

At T6, the number of retained subjects was 286, and the number of drop-outs was 87. The percentage of retention was 286/(286 + 87) = 76.6 %, and the drop-out percentage was 87/286 = 30.4 %.

At T6, the drop-out group had a higher percentage of male than the retained subjects group. The two groups did not differ significantly in other socio-demographic and psychosocial characteristics.

Biases Due to Drop-Outs

Having compared the characteristics of the retained subjects and dropped out subjects at T2–T6, what might have been the biases that were caused by sample attrition?

We found that at the earlier time points (T2, T3, and T4), drop-out groups tended to have higher percentages of subjects who were male, older, non-student, having a longer history of drug abuse, and in residential agencies at their respective previous time points. There were several possible scenarios that residential subjects at a time point became excluded from the sample at the next time point. First, these subjects might have finished their residential programmes and left before the next interview. Before they left, if they were not invited by agency staff to continue their interviews in subsequent time points, or if they did not agree to continue their participation, then these cases would be lost. Second, as explained at the beginning of Chap. 2, in the analysis of data pertaining to drug use and its socio-demographic and psychosocial correlates, subjects in residential programmes were excluded, for the reason that the drug-free status in the treatment setting was artificially achieved. Thus, if a residential subject at a time point continued to be in the programme at the next time point(s), he/she would continue to be counted as a drop-out and be left out in the data analysis.

What is important about these residential cases is that, after their departure from residential T&R programmes, whether or not they could remain drug-free, and the factors that affected their drug use/drug-free status were valuable information for comparing with non-residential subjects. Missing such data was where the major bias of the sample lied.

Fortunately, this bias diminished in the course of time, as more and more residential subjects had dropped out. As can be seen from Table 2.1, the number of subjects in residential agencies was 185 at T1, but decreased to 108 at T2, and further decreased sharply to 57 at T3, 21 at T4, 20 at T5, and 12 at T6. Thus, the negative effect of this bias was neither serious nor long-lasting.

Another indicator of possible bias in the sample was how much the retained subjects and dropped-out subjects differed in drug use in previous time points. If the two groups were significantly different in drug use, then a high drop-out rate would lead to serious bias. Fortunately, except at T2, where drop-outs were more likely than retained subjects to be drug-free at T1, the two groups did not differ significantly in drug use at all subsequent time points (see Tables 1, 2, 3, 4, and 5).

No longitudinal studies can be immunized from biases caused by sample attrition. Our analysis of the drop-out group of the sample at various time points has shown that the attrition of residential cases from the survey was perhaps the major source of bias. But fortunately, our analysis also showed that the bias was not serious and was quite limited to the sample at T2.

Lastly, a remark should be made on the selection of cases for the analysis of the influence of socio-demographic and psychosocial variables on drug use at each time point. As subjects in residential programmes were excluded (except new clients who had reported drug use in the last 30 days), the number of "retained subjects" in each sample would be smaller than the number of retained subjects indicated in Tables 1, 2, 3, 4, and 5, which included subjects of both residential programmes and outreach agencies. Strictly speaking, these were not drop-out cases. They were just cases that were not selected because they did not meet the selection criteria required for a certain analysis.

Appendix Two: Bivariate Relationships for Selection of Variables into Regression Models Testing Gender Differences

The following tables (Tables 6–17) show the bivariate correlations between drug use in the last 30 days and psychosocial variables and drug use history, and the bivariate correlations among the psychosocial variables, for the two gender groups. Independent variables that yielded significant bivariate correlations with the dependent variable concerned at four or more time points were given in *italics* in each table. These independent varaibles were chosen to be included in their respective probit regressions.

Table 6 T1–T6 bivariate correlations between drug use in the last 30 days and psychosocial variables and drug use history among males

	r					
Independent variables	T1	T2	T3	T4	T5	T6
No. of years of drug use	−.314*	−.189*	−.168*	−.019	−079	.049
Permissiveness to regular drug use	.243*	.292*	.432*	.359*	.363*	.334*
Permissiveness to occasional drug use	.432*	.418*	.351*	.272*	.279*	.245*
Disappointment if aspired education level is not achieved	−.022	−.043	.044	.008	−.087	−.132
Ever been discriminated by other people	−.153*	−.122*	−.007	.043	.032	.238*
Uncertainty about future	.033	.118*	.010	.163*	.049	.110
Think that doing extreme things shows vitality of young people	.096*	.124*	.224*	.235*	.212*	.139
Wish to have own family, job, and normal life in future	−.043	.009	−.066	−.067	−.158*	−.198*
Think that parents don't know how to teach children	.014	.035	−.003	.075	.194*	.178*
Think that school doesn't know how to teach students	.155*	.060	.145*	.005	.149*	.066
Life satisfaction	−.224*	−.284*	−.249*	−.458*	−.458*	−.212*
Self-esteem	−.038	−.076	−.141*	−.330*	−.218*	−.237*
Depression	.078	.105*	.159*	.355*	.396*	.325*
Stricken by stressful events	.065	.039	.101	.156*	.198*	.052
Subjective weathering	−.035	−.011	−.019	.106	−.134	−.044

Independent variables that yielded significant bivariate correlations with drug use in the last 30 days at four or more time points were given in *Italics*
$^*p < .05$

Table 7 T1–T6 bivariate correlations between permissiveness to regular drug use and psychosocial variables and drug use history among males

	r					
	T1	T2	T3	T4	T5	T6
No. of years of drug use	−.111*	−.037	−.074	−.165*	−.091	.019
Permissiveness to occasional drug use	.469*	.581*	.558*	.543*	.669*	.636*
Disappointment if aspired education level is not achieved	−.098*	−.196*	.051	.000	−.176*	−.135
Ever been discriminated by other people	−.096*	−.096	−.032	−.031	−.075	−.057
Sense of uncertainty about future	.029	.158*	−.021	.045	−.007	−.091
Think that doing extreme things shows the vitality of young people	.229*	.303*	.375*	.338*	.426*	.075
Wish to have own family, job, and normal life in future	−.182*	−.129*	−.209*	−.225*	−.324*	−.414*
Think that parents don't know how to teach children	.037	.031	.048	.153*	−.002	.143
Think that school doesn't know how to teach students	.119*	.077	.124*	.124	.128	−.012
Life satisfaction	−.112*	−.230*	−.063	−.141*	−.188*	.047
Self-esteem	.007	−.093	−.032	−.156*	−.085	−.053
Depression	−.001	.088	−.027	.057	.073	−.003
Stricken by stressful events	.000	−.060	.080	.009	.044	−.127
Subjective weathering	−.013	.023	−.097	.169*	−.005	−.029

Independent variables that yielded significant bivariate correlations with permissiveness to regular drug use at four or more time points were given in *Italics*
$*p < .05$

Table 8 T1–T6 bivariate correlations between permissiveness to occasional drug use and psychosocial variables and drug use history among males

	r					
	T1	T2	T3	T4	T5	T6
No. of years of drug use	−.255*	−.159*	−.156*	−.186*	−.152*	−.059
Permissiveness to regular drug use	.469*	.581*	.558*	.543*	.669*	.636*
Disappointment if aspired education level is not achieved	−.123*	−.187*	−.056	−.020	−.099	−.134
Ever been discriminated by other people	−.104*	.005	−.010	−.013	.010	.053
Sense of uncertainty about future	.038	.205*	.114	.053	.030	.085
Think that doing extreme things shows the vitality of young people	.330*	.364*	.409*	.389*	.374*	.169*
Wish to have own family, job, and normal life in future	−.126*	−.054	−.112	−.133*	−.255*	−.335*
Think that parents don't know how to teach children	.075	.117*	.189*	.180*	.138*	.149
Think that school doesn't know how to teach students	.210*	.237*	.166*	.103	.167*	.093
Life satisfaction	−.150*	−.248*	−.225*	−.248*	−.287*	−.027
Self-esteem	.051	−.097	−.021	−.133*	−.162*	−.186*
Depression	.087	.145*	.137*	.103	.194*	.189*
Stricken by stressful events	.073	.053	.163*	.064	.096	.047
Subjective weathering	−.084	.028	−.105	.004	−.047	.075

Independent variables that yielded significant bivariate correlations with permissiveness to occasional drug use at four or more time points were given in *Italics*
$*p < .05$

Table 9 T1–T6 bivariate correlations between life satisfaction and psychosocial variables and drug use history among males

	r					
	T1	T2	T3	T4	T5	T6
No. of years of drug use	.171*	.062	.077	.043	.089	−.081
Permissiveness to regular drug use	−.112*	−.230*	−.063*	−.141*	−.188*	.047
Permissiveness to occasional drug use	−.150*	−.248*	−.225	−.248*	−.287*	−.027
Disappointment if aspired education level is not achieved	−.086	.042	−.065	−.129	−.069	−.017
Ever been discriminated by other people	−.071	−.077	−.166*	−.158*	−.097	−.296*
Sense of uncertainty about future	−.194*	−.237*	−.289*	−.323*	−.157*	−.216*
Think that doing extreme things shows the vitality of young people	.042	−.131*	−.134*	−.116	−.104	−.172*
Wish to have normal life in future	.024	.078	.046	.208*	.109	.031
Think that parents don't know how to teach children	−.169*	−.190*	−.271*	−.185*	−.271*	−.304*
Think that school doesn't know how to teach students	−.127*	−.145*	−.1579*	−.009	−.231*	−.190*
Self-esteem	.289*	.387*	.364*	.531*	.395*	.431*
Depression	−.296*	−.408*	−.377*	−.531*	−.433*	−.502*
Stricken by stressful events	−.141*	−.115*	−.076	−.102	−.170*	−.131
Subjective weathering	.042	−.037	−.028	−.097	.001	−.185*

Independent variables that yielded significant bivariate correlations with life satisfaction at four or more time points were given in *Italics*

*$p < .05$

Table 10 T1–T6 bivariate correlations between self-esteem and psychosocial variables and drug use history among males

	r					
	T1	T2	T3	T4	T5	T6
No. of years of drug use	−.176*	−.125*	−.128*	.013	.060	−.114
Permissiveness to regular drug use	.007	−.093	−.032	−156*	−.085*	−.053
Permissiveness to occasional drug use	.051	−.097	−.021	−.133*	−.162	−.186*
Disappointment if aspired education level is not achieved	−.170*	−.045	−.122	−.191*	−.136	−.072
Ever been discriminated by other people	−.197*	−.149*	−.127*	−172*	−.115	−.350*
Sense of uncertainty about future	−.314*	−.172*	−.378*	−452*	−.268*	−.245*
Think that doing extreme things shows the vitality of young people	.024	−.033	−.099	−.130	−.231*	−.227*
Wish to have own family, job, and normal life in future	.093*	.118*	.098	.210*	.227*	.195*
Think that parents don't know how to teach children	−.098*	−.216*	−.140*	−.155*	−.211*	−.353*
Think that school doesn't know how to teach students	.122*	−.047	.019	−.041	−.061	−.133
Life satisfaction	.289*	.387*	.364*	.531*	.395*	.431*
Depression	−.497*	−.502*	−.560*	−.609*	−.501*	−.661*
Stricken by stressful events	−.101*	−.055	−.047	−.098	−.070	−.182*
Subjective weathering	−.188*	−.100	−.169*	−.286*	−.214*	−.262*

Independent variables that yielded significant bivariate correlations with self-esteem at four or more time points were given in *Italics*
$^*p < .05$

Table 11 T1–T6 bivariate correlations between depression and psychosocial variables and drug use history among males

	r					
	T1	T2	T3	T4	T5	T6
No. of years of drug use	.111*	.132*	.084	.126	−.004	.082
Permissiveness to occasional drug use	.087	.145*	.137*	.103	.194*	.189*
Permissiveness to regular drug use	−.001	.088	−.027	.057	.073	−.003
Disappointment if aspired education level is not achieved	.186*	−.024	.156*	.153*	.044	.109
Ever been discriminated by other people	.309*	.251*	.311*	.360*	.230*	.361*
Sense of uncertainty about future	.275*	.260*	.446*	.442*	.330*	.332*
Think that doing extreme things shows the vitality of young people	.057	.141*	.166*	.079	.093	.196*
Wish to have normal life in future	.011	−.037	.122*	−.099	−.116	−.031
Think that parents don't know how to teach children	.171*	.270*	.291*	.216*	.315*	.320*
Think that school doesn't know how to teach students	.058	.115*	.173*	.010	.242*	.223*
Life satisfaction	−.296*	−.408*	−.377*	−.531*	−.433*	−.502*
Self-esteem	−.497*	−.502*	−.560*	−.609*	−.501*	−.661*
Stricken by stressful events	.218*	.179*	.227*	.230*	297*	.321*
Subjective weathering	.130*	.070	.074	.118	.087	.211*

Independent variables that yielded significant bivariate correlations with depression at four or more time points were given in *Italics*

*$p < .05$

Table 12 T1–T6 bivariate correlations between drug use in the last 30 days and psychosocial variables and drug use history among females

	r					
Independent variables	T1	T2	T3	T4	T5	T6
No. of years of drug use	−.183*	−.126	.087	−.031	.042	.020
Permissiveness to regular drug use	.427*	.259*	.442*	.263*	.276*	.227*
Permissiveness to occasional drug use	.343*	.389*	.275*	.174*	.262*	.094
Disappointment if aspired education level is not achieved	−.037	−.009	.053	.071	.132	.178
Ever been discriminated by other people	−.063	−.074	−.012	.014	.011	.043
Sense of uncertainty about future	−.005	.088	.195*	.256*	.128	.171
Think that doing extreme things shows the vitality of young people	.167*	.122	.193*	.244*	.280*	.112
Wish to have own family, job, and normal life in future	−.120	−.161*	−.008	.116	−.021	.078
Think that parents don't know how to teach children	−.109	−.116	−.256*	.120	−.043	−.010
Think that school doesn't know how to teach students	.124*	.044	−.090	.062	.180*	.039
Life satisfaction	−.299*	−.296*	−.381*	−.260*	−.280*	−.335*
Self-esteem	−.151*	−.134*	−.210*	−.237*	−.331*	−.249*
Depression	.226*	.198*	.253*	.390*	.278*	.405*
Stricken by stressful events	.091	.095	.086	.191*	.218*	.300*
Subjective weathering	−.048	−.040	−.019	−.135	−.051	−.025

Independent variables that yielded significant bivariate correlations with drug use in the last 30 days at four or more time points were given in *Italics*

*$p < .05$

Table 13 T1–T6 bivariate correlations between permissiveness to regular drug use and psychosocial variables and drug use history among females

	r					
Independent variables	T1	T2	T3	T4	T5	T6
No. of years of drug use	−.154*	−.051	.099	−.014	−.004	.092
Permissiveness to occasional drug use	.544*	.500*	.478*	.533*	.589*	.622*
Disappointment if aspired education level is not achieved	−.154*	−.093	−.066	−.373*	−.090	−.001
Ever been discriminated by other people	−.086	−.076	−.104	−.095	−.108	.005
Sense of uncertainty about future	−.029	.076	.085	.068	.016	−.003
Think that doing extreme things shows the vitality of young people	.310*	.341*	.315*	.368*	.277*	.269*
Wish to have normal life in future	−.059	−.133	−.182*	−.103	−.237*	−.139
Think that parents don't know how to teach children	−.023	.100	−.055	.148	−.008	.149
Think that school doesn't know how to teach students	.118	.049	−.055	.055	.254*	.150
Life satisfaction	−.159*	−.182*	−.181*	−.094	−.157	−.119
Self-esteem	−.064	−.142*	−.185*	−.160*	−.214*	−.241*
Depression	.184*	.064	.190*	.171*	.114	.204*
Stricken by stressful events	.032	−.031	.024	.045	.124	.110
Subjective weathering	−.096	−.201*	−.018	−.169*	−.004	−.044

Independent variables that yielded significant bivariate correlations with permissiveness to regular drug use at four or more time points were given in *Italics*

*$p < .05$

Table 14 T1–T6 bivariate correlations between permissiveness to occasional drug use and psychosocial variables and history of drug use among females

	r					
Independent variables	T1	T2	T3	T4	T5	T6
No. of years of drug use	−.222*	−.210*	−.147	−.084	−.049	.077
Permissiveness to regular drug use	.544*	.500*	.478*	..533*	.589*	.622*
Disappointment if aspired education level is not achieved	−.230*	−.130	−.066	−.233*	−.102	.014
Ever been discriminated by other people	−.177*	−.069	−.062	−.247*	−.075	−.072
Sense of uncertainty about future	.031	.068	.395*	.242*	.100	.056
Think that doing extreme things shows the vitality of young people	.385*	.379*	.388*	.358*	.387*	.236*
Wish to have own family, job, and normal life in future	−.114	−.107	−.047	.014	−.164	−.080
Think that parents don't know how to teach children	−.057	−.084	−.074	−.090	−.041	−.019
Think that school doesn't know how to teach children	.176*	.171*	.066	−.113	.217*	.040
Life satisfaction	−.086	−.234*	−.329*	−.184*	−.066	−.047
Self-esteem	.035	−.072	−.304*	−.140	−.206*	−.228*
Depression	.045	.105	.272*	.175*	.063	.130
Stricken by stressful events	−.001	.079	.092	.001	.088	.054
Subjective weathering	−.051	−.153*	−.043	−.048	.003	−.053

Independent variables that yielded significant bivariate correlations with permissiveness to occasional drug use at four or more time points were given in *Italics*
$^{*}p < .05$

Table 15 T1–T6 bivariate correlations between life satisfaction and psychosocial variables and drug use history among females

	r					
	T1	T2	T3	T4	T5	T6
No. of years of drug use	.062	−.006	.044	−.098	.005	.124
Permissiveness to occasional drug use	−.086	−.234*	−.329*	−.184*	−.066	−.047
Permissiveness to regular drug use	−.159*	−.182*	−.181*	−.094	−.157	−.119
Disappointment if aspired education level is not achieved	−.049	−.176*	−.105	.001	−.238*	−.187*
Ever been discriminated by other people	−.129*	−.241*	−.179*	.002	.013	−.148
Sense of uncertainty about future	−.226*	−.328*	−.315*	−.299*	−.303*	−.301*
Think that doing extreme things shows the vitality of young people	−.044	−.138*	−.168*	−.122	−.050	−.076
Wish to have own family, job, and normal life in future	.016	−.043	.086	−.069	.048	.151
Think that parents don't know how to teach children	−.169*	−.173*	.005	−.288*	−.091	.072
Think that school doesn't know how to teach students	−.205*	−.287*	−.032	−.029	−.141	−.034
Self-esteem	.401*	.549*	.532*	.478*	.487*	.658*
Depression	−.461*	−.587*	−.484*	−.496*	−.576*	−.558*
Stricken by stressful events	−.077	−.262*	−.145	−.207*	−.280*	−.205*
Subjective weathering	.012	−.014	.124	−.005	−.088	−.171

Independent variables that yielded significant bivariate correlations with drug use in the last 30 days at four or more time points were given in *Italics*
$^{*}p < .05$

Table 16 T1–T6 bivariate correlations between self-esteem and psychosocial variables and drug use history among females

	r					
Independent variables	T1	T2	T3	T4	T5	T6
No. of years of drug use	.042	.014	.041	.059	.107	.112
Permissiveness to occasional drug use	.035	−.072	−.304*	−.140	−.206*	−.228*
Permissiveness to regular drug use	−.064	−.142*	−.185*	−.160*	−.214*	−.241*
Disappointment if aspired education level is not achieved	−.149*	−.136	−.180*	−.155	−.265*	−.226*
Ever been discriminated by other people	−.211*	−.132	−.143	−.096	−.028	−.192*
Sense of uncertainty about future	−.249*	−.402*	−.429*	−.360*	−.420*	−.406*
Think that doing extreme things shows the vitality of young people	−.057	−.149*	−.186*	−.195*	−.246*	−.158
Wish to have own family, job, and normal life in future	.010	−.067	.127	.036	.085	.192*
Think that parents don't know how to teach children	−.128*	−.173*	−.125	−.172*	−.118	−.074
Think that school doesn't know how to teach students	−.060	−.177*	−.163*	−.022	−.168	−.132
Life satisfaction	.401*	.549*	.532*	.478*	.487*	.658*
Depression	−.662*	−.655*	−.625*	−.663*	−.731*	−.623*
Stricken by stressful events	−.148*	−.207*	−.161*	−.082	−.139	−.136
Subjective weathering	−.080	−.109	−.026	−.001	.010	−.094

Independent variables that yielded significant bivariate correlations with self-esteem at four or more time points were given in *Italics*
*$p < .05$

Table 17 T1–T6 bivariate correlations between depression and psychosocial variables and drug use history among females

	r					
Independent variables	T1	T2	T3	T4	T5	T6
No. of years of drug use	−.119	−.030	−.053	−.042	.005	−.015
Permissiveness to occasional drug use	.045	.105	.272*	.175*	.063	.130
Permissiveness to regular drug use	.184*	.064	.190*	.171*	.114	.204*
Disappointment if aspired education level is not achieved	.188*	.141*	.275*	.106	.245*	.183
Ever been discriminated by other people	.226*	.253*	.181*	.190*	.131	.227*
Sense of uncertainty about future	.278*	.392*	.438*	395*	.394*	.383*
Think that doing extreme things shows the vitality of young people	.205*	.142*	.159*	.303*	.146	.110
Wish to have own family, job, and normal life in future	.021	.084	−.024	.082	.042	.086
Think that parents don't know how to teach children	.265*	.252*	.230*	.312*	.193*	.120
Think that school doesn't know how to teach students	.228*	.296*	.190*	.095	.291*	.286*
Life satisfaction	−.461*	−.587*	−.484*	−.496*	−.576*	−.558*
Self-esteem	−.662*	−.655*	−.625*	−.663*	−.731*	−.623*
Stricken by stressful events	.279*	.312*	.318*	.303*	.248*	.317*
Subjective weathering	−.025	.047	−.108	−.115	−.032	.010

Independent variables that yielded significant bivariate correlations with depression at four or more time points were given in *Italics*
$*p < .05$

Index

The original version of this Index was revised. The version supplied here includes final author corrections.

Y.W. Cheung, N.W.-t. Cheung, *Psychoactive Drug Abuse in Hong Kong*, Quality of Life in Asia 11, DOI 10.1007/978-981-10-6154-7

The manufacturer's authorised representative in the EU is Springer Nature Customer Service Centre GmbH, Europaplatz 3, 69115 Heidelberg, Germany. If you have any concerns regarding our products, please contact ProductSafety@springernature.com

Printed and bound by CPI Group (UK) Ltd, Croydon, CR0 4YY
25/09/2026
02222896-0016